Spirituality

Learn Reiki and Self-healing Techniques

(Discover How to Increase Your Energy, Improve Your Health and Reduce Stress)

Kathleen Lange

Published by Rob Miles

Kathleen Lange

All Rights Reserved

Spiritual Healing: Learn Reiki and Self-healing Techniques (Discover How to Increase Your Energy, Improve Your Health and Reduce Stress)

ISBN 978-1-989990-50-6

All rights reserved. No part of this guide may be reproduced in any form without permission in writing from the publisher except in the case of brief quotations embodied in critical articles or reviews.

Legal & Disclaimer

The information contained in this book is not designed to replace or take the place of any form of medicine or professional medical advice. The information in this book has been provided for educational and entertainment purposes only.

The information contained in this book has been compiled from sources deemed reliable, and it is accurate to the best of the Author's knowledge; however, the Author cannot guarantee its accuracy and validity and cannot be held liable for any errors or omissions. Changes are periodically made to this book. You must consult your doctor or get professional medical advice before using any of the suggested remedies, techniques, or information in this book.

Upon using the information contained in this book, you agree to hold harmless the Author from and against any damages, costs, and expenses, including any legal fees potentially resulting from the application of any of the information provided by this guide. This disclaimer applies to any damages or injury caused by the use and application, whether directly or indirectly, of any advice or information presented, whether for breach of contract, tort, negligence, personal injury, criminal intent, or under any other cause of action.

You agree to accept all risks of using the information presented inside this book. You need to consult a professional medical practitioner in order to ensure you are both able and healthy enough to participate in this program.

Table of Contents

INTRODUCTION 1

CHAPTER 1: THE "BIOENERGETIC" AND REIKI THERAPIES .. 4

CHAPTER 2: HOW TO ENERGIZE THE CHAKRAS 16

CHAPTER 3: REIKI FOR EVERYONE 23

CHAPTER 4: TYPES OF YOGA 54

CHAPTER 5: SOURCES OF REIKI 64

CHAPTER 6: ENERGY FLOODING WITH REIKI 80

CHAPTER 7: THE THIRD CHAKRA 95

CHAPTER 8: REIKI SELF-TREATMENT 100

CHAPTER 9: MEDITATION 102

CHAPTER 10: HOW DOES ANGELIC REIKI ENERGY WORK 109

CHAPTER 11: THE PLACE OF THE MASTER/TEACHER 115

CHAPTER 12: HOW TO PERFORM REIKI 125

CHAPTER 13: THE PRACTICE OF REIKI 134

CHAPTER 14: SOLVING PROBLEMS THE REIKI WAY 139

CHAPTER 15: HUMAN PHYSIOLOGY 142

CHAPTER 16: THE PROCESS OF ATTUNEMENT 159

CHAPTER 17: WORKING HONESTLY 165

CHAPTER 18: REIKI AND KARMA 178

CHAPTER 19: YOGA POSES FOR BEGINNERS 183

CHAPTER 20: INCLUDES AN IN-DEPTH SELF-TREATMENT MEDITATION. 190

CONCLUSION 193

Introduction

Reflection is something we as a whole ought to do all the time. Attributable to the way that we lead a riotous way of life, we as a whole need something to quiet us down and keep us stimulated, crisp, and loose. Each individual on the planet has those days during when they feel down, during which they feel like all they need to do is slither into bed and rest, which is mostly not their typical selves. There are a ton of purposes behind this sort of inclination, and these reasons may incorporate issues at work, issues with family, cash issues, and medical problems, etc. Notwithstanding, chakra contemplation is something that can enable you to dodge this inclination and make you feel all-around great once more.

There are seven chakras in your body. They are named the sun oriented plexus chakra, throat chakra, heart chakra, sacral chakra, root chakra, crown chakra, and third eye chakra. These chakras represent different things, for example, knowledge, love, sexuality, correspondence, innovativeness, etc. With the end goal for you to feel total, cheerful, and loose, the majority of your chakras must be perfect. Purging your chakras is something you ought to never disregard, as this can lead you down the way of accomplishment, wellbeing, and joy; and it can make you an entirely different individual than you were previously.

Chakra contemplation is utilized to clean your chakras and to adjust them. At whatever point you feel like there is a significant issue with you however you can't put your finger on the subject, you will profit by this sort of reflection. Through chakra contemplation, there will be a ton of advantages that will contact you and show themselves in your regular day to day existence. For example, by purging your chakras, you will begin feeling better not long after you have been doing it for a brief timeframe - some of the time even simply following a week or somewhere in the vicinity. When you first begin cleaning your chakras, you should attempt to do it consistently, or possibly three or four times each week, as this is required at the start of the purifying procedure. After some time has passed, you will presumably have the option to do it a few times per week.

More or less, chakra reflection is a sort of contemplation that will bring about cleaning your chakras and in making you feel loose, satisfied, upbeat and by and mostly better than anyone might have expected previously.

Chapter 1: The "Bioenergetic" And Reiki Therapies

Currently, a large number of therapies are being released under the label of "energy" or "bioenergetic" therapies. Such is the case of practices such as "touch for health", gem therapy or imposition of stones, a variety of spiritual healing practices, various forms of mental healing and different forms of handshakes. Many other therapies, without being directly sheltered under the classification of "bioenergetic", propose theories that attempt to explain their functioning through the incidence of supposed energies that would regulate the functioning of our personalities at different levels: physical, energetic, emotional, mental and spiritual. Among the best known we can find homeopathy, Bach flowers, and other floral remedies, as well as different elixirs of gems, planets, metals ..., radionics, chromotherapy, etc.

Given the absence of scientific data that unequivocally explain the effects observed in the application of these therapies, many of its practitioners or students seek the explanation of their effects on the knowledge that comes to us from ancient times and the philosophies of other cultures.

For better and worse, the public's great interest in these techniques has led to a large market of informative literature intended for consumption by a heterogeneous audience. Commercial interests in this regard and that of individuals who only seek social recognition and increase their business have led to much of this literature striving to give these techniques an artificially attractive aspect, omitting or falsifying certain aspects of same.

Thus many people have developed an idea about these therapies that, in many cases, does not correspond to reality. Worse, people who are introduced to the practice of these techniques are often encouraged by misconceptions that awaken false expectations and erroneous ways of acting that can lead to disappointments or other problems, being harmed them and the people who harm them. They go in search of service.

These are some of the most widespread false myths about all the referred therapies:

a)They are harmless. In many of them, it is intended that they lack side effects or that their practice lacks any risk. My vision in this regard is that everything has a dual nature, that what can help can hurt if it is applied incorrectly.

b)They offer the solution to any type of problem. Although many of these techniques can support the recovery of any problem, this does not imply that by applying only one of these techniques we can expect to have enough means to face any disruption.

c)They are scientific. Science is moving within very precise parameters and is very precise in its definitions and affirmations. For an explanation to be considered scientific it is not enough that it seems to make sense, but that it must be demonstrated under controlled environments and in a reproducible way. In fact, medicine, in general, is far from being considered scientific, despite making use of knowledge and technical means developed thanks to scientific research.

Reiki is one of the techniques that are included in this situation. It is usually considered as a form of imposition of hands; In fact, many people use the term Reiki as a synonym for the imposition of hands. Indeed, in Reiki, the imposition of hands is used for healing, especially in the 1st level of training, which this course deals with, but we must not forget that Reiki uses other techniques such as distance healing or initiations, in which there is no imposition of hands.

The first degree of Reiki acts on the "energetic" level and is aimed at restoring health on the physical and emotional levels, many people will not agree with this given the difficulty of differentiating the emotional and mental plane. The second level of Reiki deals with healing the mental plane and Reiki, in general, seeks the integration of the spiritual plane. Note that I speak of integration and fleeing the word "evolution." The evolution of the spirit will be given by experimentation, what we can do to improve this evolution is to consciously integrate the spirit into our lives, taking every day to transcendent levels and elevating our experience to the level of the spiritual.

Reiki comes from a culture in which the concept of "ki" is traditionally used to understand certain facets of the universe. Changing the word "ki" to "energy" would be too bold, but we may not have another more appropriate word in our vocabulary. Ki would be the immanent part of all things. A kind of flow that unites and finally forms the different manifestations that occur in the universe. The Rei-Ki would be "the elevated and mysterious spiritual manifestation of the universal essence". From the beginning, Reiki is conceived as a spiritual-bioenergetic therapy: spiritual because the ultimate goal is the integration of the spirit into our life and bioenergetic (serve the expression) because it works from the manipulation of that non-physical manifestation that is the Ki, the life-giving force.

Obviously, this moves Reiki away from being understandable from current science. But its effects are tangible, although not measurable, for the vast majority of people who practice it or undergo treatment. Of the truth or the false that Reiki can be, it is not I who has to pronounce, but each one has to judge and draw their own conclusions.

Reiki affects the Ki that is in us, improving it until the disease disappears but do remember that the human being is a physical manifestation in addition to spiritual, mental and "bioenergetic". Would it be sensible to expect many diseases to remit if we simply affect one of the dimensions in which the disease manifests? Should we expect a malnourished child to regain his health and grow normally only by receiving Reiki daily? If this were so, we would have found the remedy to hunger in the world. In the same way, for example, we cannot expect that a person who has renounced all his aspirations in life and submits all his acts to the approval of others will reach an emotional balance just by taking a pill. The disease usually manifests itself in multiple planes of the person, and in many cases, it is not enough to act solely on one of them to root out the disease.

It is important that we remember this aspect of the therapies to which we refer. The bioenergetic plane is one among others of those affected by the disease. By extension, this must also be applied to Reiki.

To be rigorous, Reiki directly affects not only the bioenergetic plane but also acts on the mental plane on the second and third levels. Despite this, the physical plane is not directly affected by Reiki, it is only affected to a certain extent from the transformations produced in the previous planes. If we do not support the actions of bioenergetic therapies with actions on the other planes of being, the treatment will be incomplete and will not reach the maximum of its possibilities, and, in the worst case possible, it will be useless.

In conclusion, bioenergetic therapies treat certain levels of the disease manifestation. This may be sufficient when the problem basically affects these planes, but in many cases, the disease involves several levels of manifestation in an undifferentiated manner. In these cases, it is necessary to complement these therapies with other actions that extend the treatment to those other levels involved in each case. A basic "hygiene" in the way of life is necessary.

If we consider that the human being exists in parallel in the physical, bioenergetic-emotional, mental and spiritual planes and that Reiki can only deal with the last three, in each case we must consider the need to apply techniques that act on the physical plane (diet, chiropractic, exercise, hygiene, phytotherapy, etc.). In addition, for the first and second grade, we will remember that there are other levels of manifestation of the person and the disease (mind) that may need extra support.

Focusing on the first level of Reiki, the object of this manual, the objective pursued by the practice of the system at this level is the self-healing of the student, especially in aspects that affect the physical and emotional levels. Since a disharmony manifested in, for example, the mental plane can be reflected psychically or spiritually, it is necessary that the first-degree Reiki practitioner has tools that allow him to stop or alleviate the evils rooted in those planes outside the scope of his level Reiki if you intend to reach an important level of self-healing.

This is reflected in the information we have about Reiki primitive schools. In addition to the practice of Reiki, students were indoctrinated about the importance of nutrition (physical plane), ethics and philosophy (mental plane). This was linked to the direct action of Reiki on the bioenergetic and emotional planes, covering the entire spectrum of manifestation of our existence. From that moment on, the person assumes his responsibility in the maintenance or recovery of his state of health, applying and developing the means obtained for this purpose.

We must not understand that the first level Reiki practitioner is a self-sufficient person, who does not need other people to solve their health problems. As one person says to me that I consider "the dentist does not remove his own teeth". In many cases, the diseases are well-rooted and all help is little to eradicate them.

Chapter 2: How To Energize The Chakras

Chakra centers are stimulated everyday through the physical senses or thoughts. Human beings energize their centers, either unconsciously or consciously, through different ways.

Energizing Through Thoughts

Positive thoughts have been proven by science to allow a person's energy to flow unrestricted and freely. On the other hand, negative thoughts are said to decrease the body's energy. Every emotional or mental thought is associated with a chakra. For example, an angry thought is said to lower the flow of red energy while a passionate thought increases it. This means that if you are continuously angry, you will reduce the energy of your root chakra.

Energizing Through the Sun

As the most significant source of energy, the Sun gives energy to human beings, plants, animals, water, and even the chakras. The sunlight allows all the color energies to flow to the Earth.

Energizing Through Food

Sunlight provides energy to plants. The color energy stays in the plant through its flower, vegetable, or fruit. This energy provides nutritional value to any person who consumes the plant. Thus, by eating food which contains any of the color energies, the chakras in the body are also balanced.

Energizing Through Visualization

Thought as an energy can maintain the chakra centers through breathing, visualization, and meditation exercises.

The vibration of the chakra becomes more powerful when color intention is added.

Energizing Through Minerals and Gems

Minerals and gems also have energies. Crystals have similar crystalline structure like the human beings. Unknown to a lot of individuals, crystals can be programmed and can provide more power to energies. A person can wear a gem jewelry or place minerals and gems within their environment to absorb their healing vibrations.

Energizing Through Color Bathing

Since color is energy and energy is conducted through water, a person can lie in colored water in order to absorb the vibration frequency of the color. The chakra can also be balanced by thinking of the end result from the energy. Aromatherapy oil can also be added in the water. It is advisable to use organic color and not chemical food coloring.

Energizing Through Aromatherapy

Essential oils come from a flower or plant. Oil is associated to a color because it has healing properties. Quality therapeutic oils must be used because inexpensive ones may have toxins. Furthermore, oils are never directly applied to the skin. They are best diluted in a bath or with carrier oil.

Energizing Through Music and Dance

Music can affect you either in a positive or negative way. Each note is associated to a chakra center and color. There are particular sounds which can stimulate a spiritual, physical, mental, or emotional response. For example, the physical body can be energized by the beating of the drums and can stimulate the root chakra.

Energizing Through Toning and Sounds

The body is capable of creating vibrating sounds which has the same frequency as the different organs. As such, regular toning is needed to help the organs function properly. Because noise pollution can be quite disturbing, it is best for you to surround yourself with happy sounds to help with being more productive.

Energizing Through Color Tones

Different colors can be filtered to the body through shining of light. The color vibration can be absorbed by the skin and go through the chakra.

Energizing Through Solar-charged Water

Water can be charged by the sun's rays. A colored, unleaded glass is filled with water and exposed to the sun's rays or a colored filter can be used in a glass of water so that the rays can interact with the color energy.

Energizing Through Syntonics

Syntonics makes use of the eyes to stimulate the color and affect the pituitary gland in order to release hormones associated with an organ with the same frequency. There are therapeutic eyeglasses with different colored filters to boost particular chakra energy. The wearer must ensure that the eyeglasses are 100% UVA and UVB coated. Furthermore, the choice of color tint is very important.

Energizing Through Decors

The conscious use of colors in the work environment or home can also provide productive and positive energy. It is good to use various colored pillows, carpets, artworks, etc. The right color can also be used to paint a room.

Energizing Through Clothing

Clothing can also influence a person's energy level, mind, and mood. The color energy can be amplified if light is allowed to penetrate through the clothes. Furthermore, vibrant colors in clothes can facilitate better transfer of energy.

Energizing Through Art and Color

Art and colors are outlets which can be used to stimulate or express. A person must surround themselves with suitable colors. Calming colors can be used in the bedroom while stimulating colors can be used at the workplace.

Chapter 3: Reiki For Everyone

10.1. Reiki for Women

Women are the ones who encounter more problems than men. There are many working women and naturally their workload is more. After doing work in the office, they have to take care of the family and do household chores also. Women particularly encounter these types of problems.

10.1.1 Depression

For overcoming depression, women should keep one hand on the heart and the other hand on the stomach and thus pass energy. The energy from the hand goes into the heart and dissolves the blockages and women can feel better. The heartbeat slows down when you do this by 3 beats per minute. For example, the heartbeat comes down to 69 beats per minute from normal level of 72 and also the expansion of the lungs comes down to 11 from the normal level of 18 breaths per minute. Also the need for oxygen comes down since the lungs breathe slowly. The tension also comes down since the secretion of lactate in the blood comes down. It is only when the level of the lactate in blood goes up that tension arises. The lactate is secreted in the muscles of the skull. When people practise placing of hands on heart, healing starts and tension comes down. People can more relax since their hearts get Reiki energy. It gives **"relaxation response"** which is the opposite of **"FIGHT OR FLIGHT RESPONSE".** People feel more relaxed and more at ease and they fall asleep in less time.

10.1.2. Medicine of the Future

Man gets energy from food, air, water and Reiki energy. When the Reiki Energy does not go to the heart's energy centre, the heart develops problems like depression. The Reiki solution to this is to just keep your hand on the heart and say a prayer. Within a short span of time, there will be some improvement. In this method, we do not take any medicine but only energy, which is the medicine of the future. The whole of humanity should use this medicine, which is available in abundance in the cosmos. When people keep the hand on the heart, they automatically extract Reiki energy. It is a pure form of energy and hence called energy of love. Also, you don't have to pay for it. The mother uses love energy to pat the child. It is available from the almighty to everyone.

10.1.3. How can Relationship in the Family be improved?

Blessing the other person can easily solve the relationship problems. By blessing, we mean supplying the Reiki energy. Think about a person and project the Reiki energy. You can do this by keeping the hand on the heart and saying, "Let the relationship be alright". We thereby send thought wave to the other person. Suppose, the relationship is strained between husband and wife, father and son, mother and daughter, between brothers and between sisters. The same principle can be applied, i.e. projecting energy of love. It may be that at one point, you would have hurt the other person, or the other person would have hurt you. If you project good energy, i.e. a good thought, (the thought wave is electro magnetic and travels even faster than the speed of light, i.e. 3 lakh km per second), it reaches the other person and makes changes in him and he in turn projects the positive energy realizing, "Oh! I have hurt the other person and the mistake is on my part". Hence the communication is established between two hearts. This makes both of them to come together. What we have to do is to project the energy patiently for some time until the relationship is healed. The love energy will definitely unite them together.

10.1.4. How to get promotion?

Love energy means the Reiki energy. With love, we can encompass the whole world. Only love and nothing but love does the change. Love should come from the heart without any strings attached. The same principle can be extended to any activity, any relationship problem, and any situation in life. This can also be adopted to achieve goals in life. You can project the Reiki energy to your goal by saying an affirmation, "I want to get a good promotion in my office". The pre-requirement is that you should have executed work properly to the satisfaction of superiors in the office. You project this energy to your boss and continue this till goals are achieved.

10.2. How to become a No.1 Student using Reiki

This Reiki programme helps student to particularly overcome depression and examination fear by improving memory power and concentration and in healing minor ailments, etc.

10.2.1. Reiki for students

The different problems faced by the student community are 1. Lack of memory power
2. Lack of concentration
3. Sports Injuries
4. Examination fear
5. Failure to establish rapport

6. Lack of self-confidence
7. Eye strain

8. Lack of logical thinking

Let us give solutions to all the problems faced by the present-day students one by one.

10.2.2. Memory power

Memory power is required for students writing the examination. First you should understand how the lack of memory power arises. The brain is the main organ for memory. We have to activate the brain for a better memory power. In Reiki we use energy to activate the brain. When I say brain, I mean the right and left sides of the brain. We also use the visualization and affirmation techniques besides passing Reiki energy. That's why this system is very effective. For memory power, the students have to keep the two hands on the right and left sides of the brain. When you keep the hands, you automatically tap the Reiki energy from the universe. Because the intention is there to activate the brain, energy follows thought. At the same time you can give an affirmation that "My memory power has improved" and also visualize that you are getting good marks in the examination, or you are getting a prize from the principal of the college. By this, we are energizing the brain and all the neurons in the brain get activated, and face becomes bright. Memory power will improve.

Students have to practise this for a minimum of 15 minutes in the morning and evening. This can be done at any place, either in the college, or in the house. The Reiki energy flows when you keep the hand on the area. If you do not have any time, you can also do it while you are studying. For example you keep one hand on head and keep reading your book and also do this even when you are lying on the bed. When you sit in class you can keep one hand on head and do your writing. In this method, there is no time and space restriction. That's why this will be effective for improving the memory power. For many students, the memory power has improved after they practised this regularly.

10.2.3. Lack of Concentration
This is a widespread problem faced by many students. They are not able to concentrate and there are many distractions. When they are studying, many thoughts come and interfere. For concentration power, we have to further activate the pituitary gland. The pituitary gland is in the forehead. Keep the hand on the forehead and on the back head. When the forehead is activated, the pituitary gland gets charged. The pituitary gland, which is called master gland, secretes 10 types of hormones. The face becomes bright, clarity of thinking improves and you

will be able to concentrate better. Everything comes by practice only. Hence practise, practise and practise!

10.2.4. Examination Fear

The stress and tension during examination time are common for all. The common denominator in Reiki for all these problems is to keep the hands on the affected part and do visualization and affirmation. The stresses are of two types; one is an emotional stress, and another is mental stress. For emotional stress, we have to keep one hand on the heart and the other hand on the stomach, just above the navel. The energy goes to the heart and stomach, which are the emotional centres. When the energy reaches the area, the fear goes. Reiki energy releases the blockage. At the same time we should visualize, "We have become normal". Regarding mental stress, 'mental' means the brain. The afflicted student has to keep the hand on the head and pass the energy until the tension is released. When you keep the hand, the warmth in the hand opens the blood vessels and blood circulation improves. The secretion of lactate comes down. The more the secretion of lactate, more will be tension level. So when you keep your hand, tension comes down. When the tension level comes down, students can feel calm with, their heads becoming light.

During examination time, students do not get good sleep due to stress. For this too, students can keep their hands on the heart and the stomach. Prayers can be recited if they feels like it.

10.2.5. How to establish rapport?

The other important problem faced by the student is facing people. When you are meeting someone, you have to establish a rapport with him. The student can match his energy field with that of the other person. When the energy level matches, student is at the same wavelength as the other person. Before this, the student has to get rid of nervousness. For calmness and peace of mind, he has to keep the hand on the heart and the stomach. If he practices for five days, palpitation and nervousness will go away and he will remain calm and quiet. Matching the energy field comes by matching posture, breath and the voice. Suppose the person other is sitting cross-legged, he can also sit cross-legged. If he is talking in a high pitch, he should also talk in high pitch. So (aura) the energy field is matched. Whatever you say, he will say yes, yes. First cater to his interest and secondly match your energy field and then he will agree to whatever you say. Then whatever you tell, he will also be in agreement. By establishing rapport in this manner, for example, you an even get your sales contract!

10.2.6. To improve Self-confidence

Many students do not have faith in themselves. They feel that they are inferior. This may be due to the past trauma they had in their school days or college days or at home, childhood abuse etc. This trauma would be remaining in their subconscious mind. Passing the Reiki energy and giving affirmations that "my entire trauma has gone" and "I have become a better person" can remove this. If they practice this for three days, the past trauma or childhood memory will easily disappear and students will feel confident again.

10.2.7. Logical thinking

Some students are confused and are not able to think coherently. For example, if a businessman makes a wrong decision, he loses money. Clarity of thinking is a must for anybody. "A sound mind in a sound body" goes the saying. First, the body has to be in good condition. For that we have to activate the energy centres in the body. We have seen earlier the activating of the top energy centre, the forehead energy centre and the heart and stomach centres. We are now left with other three energy centres, which are important, viz. the throat energy centre, water centre and physical energy centre. The thyroid and parathyroid glands are in throat. The student has to keep the hand on the throat, front and back, and do a visualization and affirmation and activate the thyroid gland.

The other two important centres are the water centre and the root centre at the back of the spine. The end of the spine is the physical energy centre. Keep the hand on the water centre (2" below the navel) and the other hand on the base of the spine. So if you activate all seven centres, students can become hale and hearty. For logical thinking and clarity of thinking, you have to concentrate on the forehead where you have the intuitive centre. So if you activate the forehead and the back head, clarity of thinking will result because pituitary gland starts secreting all hormones properly at right quantity.

Some students do not have a practical thinking since the backside of head is blocked. He may start many projects and leave them in the middle and may not complete anything. These types of people should concentrate more on the back of the head to improve the practical thinking. The logical thinking and the practical thinking lead to positive thinking and proactive thinking.

10.3. How can one take care of his well being in day-to-day activities using Reiki?

The answer is two-fold:
1. It is easy to learn Reiki
2. It can be practised at any time.

For example, while doing your work, just keep your hand on the heart or the part of the body and automatically this energy flows into the body. Your energy field gets stabilized and no disease will affect you.

10.3.1. Not a Placebo Effect

During the course of our mission in the service of mankind, we have found that these types of techniques are very useful. First it changed me and I thought I should give the benefit of this knowledge to other people. It is really simple and effective. Afterwards, when I started helping people, I found it working very well. Lot of people has seen the proof of it.

For example, if you buy an insurance policy, it is only paper. If you buy a cassette, you get something. A doctor gives a pill. When you get give anything tangible, people are sceptical. Once you try to harness the power within yourself, you will like it.

10.3.2. Energy causes Transformation

People have been so far used to taking medicines. So, to cater to that need also, I sometimes give glucose tablets for psychological reasons. It is basically sugar. When people like me give something, patients believe it. This is only for creating a psychological impact. The Reiki energy causes the transformation.

The electrical energy flowing from the hand causes chemical change and rearranges atoms. The hands are powerful instruments available for everybody. When the energy centres are blocked due to the stresses and strains in day-to-day life, we can to clear them by simply keeping our hands on our bodies. It is only natural that some people involve religion or any other superstitious belief in this. I am practising this, however, only as a science.

10.3.3. Self-actualization needs

Maslow's Theory of self-actualization states that the man, after satisfying the physical needs, security needs and ego needs, wants to have a good self-esteem. Then afterwards he wants to utilize his fullest potential. For this it is the only easy, effective and safe method to make changes in him for becoming a successful person.

10.3.4. Results are important, name does not matter

The name or the way of the system or its discipline is not important; the results are the only things that count. Any system that works should produce results. It does not matter what the system is called or how it works. The brain is the biggest pharmaceutical industry on the earth.

Many trainers have lectured much on the physical and psychological side. But what is missing in some of the methods is the energy principle. Many scientists are and have been the recipients of Reiki Revelation.

Reiki uses Reiki Energy Principle and man's connection to it. Reiki strives to generate the positive and vital feelings of Love, Compassion, Harmony and Brotherhood in the world.

10.4. Reiki energy for stress management

Human beings encounter stress daily, be at home or at the workplace. Stress should be managed efficiently; otherwise it will lead to many diseases. Reiki energy is a very effective method for managing stress. You have only to spare some time daily and practise. You can integrate Reiki energy with your lifestyle. Then it will do wonders. We must project Reiki energy through the hands along with a good intention for it to work.

Stress often leads to heart disease. You can channel energy to the heart centre and heal. The heart is very sensitive. Do not give energy directly to heart, but give to heart chakra. If heartbeat is normal, you can directly touch the heart. When a person gets a heart attack, energy should not be directly given to heart. You can give energy to stomach and slowly it will go to heart.

10.4.1. A panacea for everything

Reiki energy dissolves everything which creates tension, unpleasantness and fatigue. We can achieve our goals and ambitions using Reiki energy. Reiki energy helps to increase the energy and creative power. The blockage in physical, mental and emotional levels is eliminated, thereby increasing the resistance to diseases. Our overall personality will improve which in turn will reflect on health and quality of life. Reiki energy is divine energy, which can heal animals, plants, and the world too.

10.5. Reiki for Sportsman
Sportsmen have to keep their body fit and healthy so that they can perform well in sports. Players have to take care of not only their body but also mind since concentration is required for success. If Reiki is practised regularly, they possess have healthy body, mind and spirit.

Allopathy deals only the symptoms of the disease whereas Reiki heals the root cause of the disease. Reiki is a Holistic system which means healing takes place at the mind, body and spirit level.

Reiki can relieve the anxiety and stress often encountered by sportsmen. The actual interpretation of stress is excessive secretion of adrenaline from adrenaline glands. A reasonable amount of adrenalin is required to produce drive for facing life. If it exceeds some limit, it is dangerous to the body. Body becomes too resistant and we get headache, hypertension, anger, irritability etc. Reiki energy relaxes the mind.

Reiki dissolves everything which creates tension, unpleasantness and fatigue. We can achieve our goals and ambitions using Reiki. Reiki helps to increase the energy and creative power. The blockage in physical, mental and emotional levels are eliminated, thereby increasing the resistance to diseases. Our overall personality will improve which in turn reflect on health and quality of life.

First aid using Reiki can be given till the patient is taken to hospital.

Other common ailments encountered by sportsmen are disc problems, backache, and disc slip, cervical, Spondlytis, muscle pain and joint Pain. These problems can be overcome if Reiki is practised regularly. Stress and a disease-free body can enable sportsmen to perform well in sports. Reiki also aids allopathy treatment thereby hastening the healing process. For mental depression and neurological disorders, Reiki is the best remedy. If tranquilizers, anti-depressants are taken, it worsens the situation rather than helping recovery. There is an instrument called Gigatens which is a battery operated instrument. It supplies the same energy as Reiki energy but it is not as effective as the element of touch is absent. Touch sense is very important and as you touch a human being, a minor volt of electricity is transferred that shoots the neurons in the brain which triggers the manufacture of neuro chemicals.

The brain is a huge factory which produces hormones which give us moods and feelings. If you are in good mood, good hormones are produced by brains which are accepted by all the cells in the body. Hence you feel happy. If you are in a unhappy situation, bad hormones are secreted which makes you feel unpleasant.

Hence there is a body & mind connection. A sound mind in sound body will follow if Reiki is channeled.

10.6. Reiki for Old People

Old people should possess with them the knowledge and remedies for staying healthy. They face problems like sense of helplessness, fear of ageing and ailments. Practising Reiki daily can rejuvenate them and strengthen their roles as parents and grandparents. Ageing often deteriorates the immune system and makes them susceptible to disease. Eighty-five percent of those over sixty-five have at least three chronic ailments. Fatigue or lack of energy can zap one's enthusiasm for life and create boredom and indifference to family. Reiki can help old persons feel better and relieve many problems.

Men gets energy not only from the food he eats, water he drinks, air he breathes but also from Reiki energy. If Reiki energy does not go into the human body, the particular area will be weak resulting in manifestation of disease.

Other common ailments are arthritis, diabetes, and stomach problem and memory loss. Arthritis is inflammation of the joints which can reduce by natural production of cortisone from adrenals. People often take cortisone supplements to relieve pain. Reiki energy can stimulate the adrenals to produce cortisone thereby reducing or eliminating pain. If Reiki energy is given to pancreas, diabetes can be controlled. For memory loss, Reiki can also stimulate the brain and remove blocked energy thereby improving blood circulation. Brain activity and memory will improve. Senior citizens can learn Reiki and improve their outlook and approach towards life.

10.7. Reiki for Managers

Reiki Healing using Universal Life Force energy is an effective technique for managers for coping with stress and improving the quality of life. When stress is not handled properly, the body's defence systems breakdown and they become more susceptible to illness and disease. Managers should have the ability to handle difficult situations. Reiki can be very practised even in the workplace by just placing the hands on the body while doing work.

Reiki dissolves everything which creates tension, unpleasantness and fatigue. We can achieve our goals and ambitions using Reiki. Reiki helps to increase the energy and creative power. The blockage in physical, mental and emotional levels are eliminated, thereby increasing the resistance to diseases. Our overall personality will improve which in turn reflect on health and quality of life.

10.8. Reiki Energy for World Peace

In the recent past, there has always been a threat of war between countries. Biological and nuclear weapons produce tension, unrest among people. War goes on between America and Iraq, Palestinians and Israelis, the South Koreans and North Koreans, India and Pakistan etc. All these things clearly indicate people are not at ease between themselves and the inner ecology is not good. Hence the outer ecology becomes bad which causes natural calamities all over the world, like storms, earthquakes, tornadoes, etc.

The need of the hour is to bring out the ecological balance. The natural balance itself is destroyed because the inner ecology is destroyed. Hence it is reflected in the outer ecology. The pollution from the automobiles and the industries bring a lot of havoc to the ozone layer in the atmosphere. These problems are created by the greedy nature of man and unwillingness of industrialists to invest in environment-friendly technologies. People do not have value for human life; have no consideration and respect for others.

All these things finally result in nature's fury. People should understand, Reiki energy has come into the world to mitigate the sufferings of human beings. Everybody is talking of Reiki energy because of the simplicity and effectiveness. For all the diseases, the only one treatment is to keep your hands. So people should be prepared to face the millennium by learning the new technique and practise it for all the dayto-day problems, i.e. physical, mental or emotional problems.

The quality of life will definitely change. There will be inner harmony, harmony in home, in the neighbourhood, in the society, in the states, in the country and between countries. If Reiki energy is practised by at least 10% of world population, there will definitely be an improvement in the overall situation of the world. For mankind, Reiki energy is a personal transformation tool. You can merge your bio-magnetism with that of the universal magnetism. Hence if you align your energy field to the universal magnetism, you can have a joyful, blissful and successful life.

The dictionary definition of Healing is hale, hearty and whole. Hence Reiki system is holistic system. Reiki attacks not only the symptoms of diseases but also the causes and works at the cellular and molecular level. That is why the man gets completely transformed from mental and physical blockages. Reiki is beyond religion, sex, nationality, languages, caste. Anybody can follow the system irrespective of creed or dogma. If people learn and practise Reiki, there will not be any problem in the world.

In today's world, fight goes on between religions, castes and regions. Reiki starts from the individual. First the individual gets transformed and then he can heal his family, society and world. Hence the famous saint Avvaiyar says "When the bund of the paddy field rises, water level rises. If the water level rises, paddy height rises. If the paddy height rises, citizens' life style rises. If citizen like style rises, the kingdom will flourish". Reiki is the universal life force. Reiki can be used for world peace by beaming Reiki energy to all leaders of the world.

After getting healed, the individual can extend its benefit to his family, to society and to the world. For example in a house there may be difference of opinion between husband and wife, father and son, between friends and relatives. If you learn and practise Reiki, these strained relationships can be healed. Likewise, if we project Reiki energy to all problems of the world with love, we can solve anything. That's why we call Reiki as "universal love force". By Reiki, we can unite the people of the whole world together. Maharishi Mahesh Yogi, Founder of Transcedental

Meditation says that if one percent of the people in the sea shore practice meditation, then there will be world peace among all the nations in the world. Reiki is the most effective and simple system.

Chapter 4: Types Of Yoga

Before one start practicing yoga, he should know which yoga is appropriate for him considering all the aspects. However, taking up a branch of yoga will not separate you from others. It is interlinked and overlapping of these practices can be seen at many places.

☐Raja yoga – This is practiced following strictly the 8 limbs of yoga by Patanjali. Here the focus is kept more on meditation.

☐ Karma yoga – This branch talks about the effect of past on the present, whereby we tend to do our best today in order make the future positive and happy. It is about self-transcending actions. Staying selfless in all aspects of life is the basic which helps to attain what we want.

☐ Bhakti yoga – As the name describes, this is about the devotional means which helps us to accept and tolerate everything that we encounter. This path deals in channelizing our emotions in order by controlling our heart. In short this is yoga of heart.

☐ Jnana yoga – This being the yoga of mind helps in attaining the wisdom/sage. By intellectually developing our mind, it is the most direct form of yoga. It is also considered to be the most difficult form. This requires studying the yogic literatures and scripts.

☐ Tantra yoga – This is the most mystical of all the other branches, as this concentrates to rituals and also includes sanctified sexuality. In this practice we find divine in all the activities one perform.

☐ Ashtanga yoga – This is the most widely known and followed branch. Ashtanga means eight limbs, which gives us the path to follow to lead a significant life ethically and morally

Warm up

Warm ups or preparatory movements are essential before you start doing the yoga asana and poses. These are the simple positions that help our muscles to stretch and relax. In simple words it can be called as warm up exercises as it gives flexibility to our body to take up all the efforts and strain.

Exercise 1:

Balance yourself, keeping the legs apart with about 1-1.5 feet distance between them and hands straight beside your body, with palms on the thighs. Look straight. (Hence forth called as pre-position)

Now slowly inhale and raise both the hands upwards keeping them parallel to each other, while maintaining some distance between them. Then, bring your hands down while exhaling slowly, and place them on your knees respectively.

Inhaling, start bending down towards ground at waist keeping the spine straight and head pressed towards knees.

Exhaling, get back to normal position.

Exercise 2:

Take pre-position. Then, inhaling slowly, raise hands till shoulders in sideways keeping them parallel to ground.

Now exhaling, bend forward at your waist. Keeping the right hand straight, touch the right foot thumb with left hand. Do not bend at the joints.

Inhaling, go back to preposition.

Do the same exercise exhaling with right hand touching left foot.

Inhaling, go back to preposition.

Exercise 3:

Take pre-position. Then, inhaling slowly, raise hands till shoulders in sideways keeping them parallel to ground.

Now exhaling, stretching as much as possible, and twist and turn the waist towards left taking your hand in the same level as they are in now.

Inhaling, get back to preposition.

Again exhaling, twist and turn towards right side now, with hands on the same position. Stretch maximum.

Inhaling, get back to preposition.

Exercise 4:

Taking preposition, inhale while you bring your hands and keep it on the waist with fingers on front and thumb back.

Keeping legs straight, exhale and bend forward at waist with head straight in line with knee position.

Inhaling, get back to pre-position.

Again exhale and bend backward as much as possible. Don't overdo and lose your balance.

Inhaling, get back to preposition.

Repeat the same action by bending sideways also. First left, then right side.

Exercise 5:

Keeping both hands on the waist, bend the neck forwards till the chin meets the pit below Adam's apple.

Slowly get back to normal position.

Now backward as much as possible without hurting yourself.

Slowly come back to normal position.

Repeat the same action by bending sideways also. First left then right side.

Exercise 6:

Standing straight, lift your left leg bending the knee to a 90 degree angle.

Hold the leg at thigh tight, stand straight and rotate the foot of the leg in clockwise and anticlockwise directions, like making a circle).

Slowly keeping the leg on ground, come back to normal position.

Now repeat the same action with right leg and complete the circle movement.

Exercise 7:

Standing straight, bend left hand elbow and to an angle of 90 degree. Keep the elbows straight and close to body.

With the help of right hand fingers catch the left hand wrist lightly, then rotate left hand in clockwise and anti-clockwise direction.

Now get back to normal position.

Repeat the same action with another hand. i.e. holding the right hand with left hand fingers and rotating right hand clockwise and anticlockwise.

Exercise 8:

Stand in preposition with hands raised up front side, keeping them parallel to ground in the level of shoulders.

Now inhaling, raise both the heels.

Exhaling, sit on the toes slowly, keeping the knees and toes pointed in the same direction.

Inhaling, slowly stand up straight.

Exhaling, get back to preposition.

Precautions:

Do all the movements slowly and smoothly.

Do not swing around or give jerks.

Let the movements be in line with your breathing.

Breathing rules

The breathing rules for each asana are specific and different from others. But generally these rules are to be kept in mind while performing yoga.

Get back to normal breathing tune when no movement is performed.

Few asanas require us to hold breath for a while. In these cases, people with breathing irregularities should not hold their breath. Instead of stretching an asana and holding it, we can repeat the same asana a few number of times to avoid difficulties. Also remember not to hold breath for longer time than required.

Chapter 5: Sources Of Reiki

Working with your own energy to start, will most definitely help you become proficient in the experience of Energy manipulation. Unfortunately your own energy is fairly finite. If you start projecting your own energy out into the world around you, you will soon start to feel drained and tired.

When Reiki is practiced to full effect, the experience of working with Reiki should be rejuvenating. This is because you do not have to use your own Reiki energy (life force). You are fully integrated and connected to an entire universe of Energy.

You can draw from this universe and project it through you. If you are having trouble with this concept, think of it like you are plugging yourself into the universal energy like a wire into a wall socket. Draw through the wire. Multiple wires if you like.

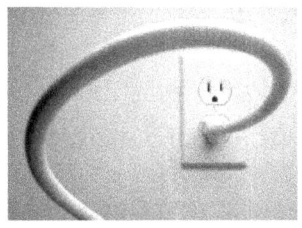

I have also had success with creating (visualizing) and connecting to the universe using a spider web / umbrella like structure. Each line catching and drawing the flow of universal energy towards me. There is no right or wrong way. Just find what works for you.

Draw (gather) energy from the air around you, the clouds and even the wind. Avoid drawing energy from the ground underneath your feet. The earth serves as an energy filter and converter. It is best to avoid drawing unfiltered energy from the earth into and through you. This may cause discomfort and even injury.

Some Energy Manipulation exercises

There are several exercises that you can perform regularly to improve your own abilities.

I have found Thai Chi particularly valuable. Not only does it considerably improve mental ability, it also incorporates various forms of energy movement practices, including working with energy balls, catching and releasing Energy. It is fun to do and will significantly enhance your abilities to focus and manipulate energy.

If you are looking to just practice your energy movement skills, visualize and create an energy ball. Resize it. Move it around. Absorb it back. Play with it...

You can also practice simple directional flow and general control exercises using the techniques described to introduce you to your first Reiki transmission.

One of the most fun ways to practice is to do so with a partner. Positioning yourself opposite your partner, create a circle with your arms by touching your palms together with your partners' palms. Push and pull is fun. Also transmit directionally. Have your partner identify which side is pushing energy, left or right. You will be surprised how rewarding it can be, especially when your partner is able to correctly identify which side is which. Verifiable evidence of your ability to manipulate Energy.

When you are ready

As a Reiki practitioner, your purpose is to heal another by providing universal Energy to aid that person's energy structures towards harmonization. This process is a very invasive process. You are working on the very essence of that person.

When you transmit Energy (Reiki) through you to another person, you should take care to transmit what you receive. No less and no more.

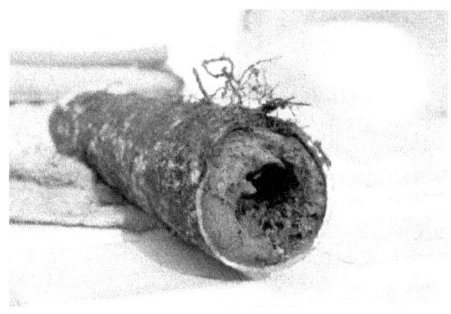

What you transmit can be contaminated by you. If you are holding thoughts other than pure intent to heal, those thoughts will be transmitted along with the healing energy you are sending. They are contaminants and will have a direct impact on the clients and their overall wellbeing.

When contaminated thoughts are imbued with emotions, they are potentially very significant. Impacts from those thoughts on your clients will prove even more substantial and disruptive to their wellbeing.

Living a healthy and balanced life will aid in your ability to deliver uncontaminated and more powerful healing to your client. By virtue of the connection of everything, as the Reiki practitioner, how you treat yourself will directly affect your Reiki practice.

Mental exercises like meditation are useful to reduce through flow of energetic contamination.

Simple breathing exercises like breath counting are particularly useful to help you learn mental focus and control.

Mindfulness and Mental Connections

A well developed ability to create strong connections between you and your client will be especially helpful to successfully deliver treatments. There are several very useful techniques for doing this effectively, however, creating these connections come with a certain level of practitioner responsibility and risk.

It is just as easy to deliver harm as it is to deliver treatment. If great care is not taken, you can easily negate the benefits of any treatments you deliver and even cause harm.

When you have created a connection between yourself and a client, you have opened high frequency multidirectional channels between yourself and your client. These channels will directly channel not only the energy you are transmitting but also convey any attitudes, feelings and emotional states that you may hold directly into the client's subconscious and energy systems. If you are feeling negative about something in your life, you will pass that feeling on to your client.

When planning a treatment, it would be wise to spend some time on self preparation. Be mindful of your own state of mind. Take steps to mitigate those feelings, establishing a sense of peace and detachment from your feelings.

Create a state of mind that is conducive to avoiding harm including using techniques like meditation, breathing exercises (e.g. breath counting), mind clearing exercises (e.g. blue light visualization) and affirmations.

You want to create a state of mental detachment from self and singular focus on purpose. This will enhance your treatment ability considerably and ensure that you only deliver clean healing.

Visualizing for success

The stronger your focus on purpose becomes, the more potent your delivery will be. Taking advantage of proven methods to focus your efforts will yield spectacular results.

One of the most potent ways of focusing the mind is visualization. Keep it simple though. Your purpose is to use the visualization as a tool, not do visualization for the sake of visualization itself.

Visualize the connection, the flow of energy, and how the energy flows through you to the client. You can also visualize ways to collect energy. There is no need to get elaborate with your visualizations. The intent is merely to focus your mind on the action you are taking.

You can use visualization as a means to construct protection for yourself. (More about that later on.)

Reiki Symbols

When using visualization, depending on your lineage, there are several traditional Reiki symbols that you can use to help focus your mind and treatment efforts. A symbol imbued with your thoughts of purpose will not only serve to focus your mind considerably but aid the successful delivery of a treatment.

In Free Flow Reiki simplicity is key. Easy to remember and connect with symbols, will make it possible for you to focus on the purpose rather than the visualization of an elaborate symbol. Whatever symbols you use, keep in mind that the symbol is a tool and is only as powerful as your use of it.

Free Flow - First Degree Symbol

The first symbol that you can use to enhance your treatments is a "spiral vortex".

{spins anti-clockwise}

{Northern Hemisphere}

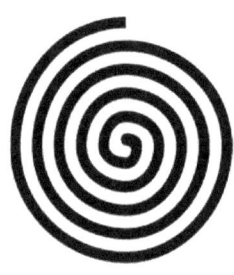

{---OR---}

{spins clockwise}

{Southern Hemisphere}

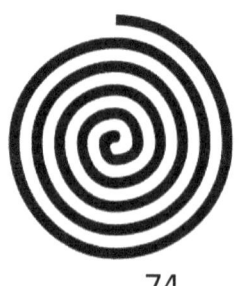

{simple representation of the "spiral vortex" symbol}

Vortices collect and deliver whatever they collect, through the bottom of the vortex. In your visualization you want the vortex to spin in the same direction as water would spin running into a drain. (Different in northern and southern hemispheres of earth as depicted in the images above)

To use the symbol you can simply visualize it with the spout pointing towards the area of treatment and the open end taking energy you deliver and funneling (pushing) it directly towards your client.

You can use this symbol to collect universal energy from around you.

You can visualize this in full color or black & white as depicted here. Make it spin at whatever speed you need to deliver the energy to the client. You can visualize this in any size that you need.

When using this symbol, project it as if coming from the palms of your hands. Energy is drawn through you and funneled directly towards the client.

You can funnel energy, light and anything else you need to pass to a client easily using this symbol to help focus your mind on delivery.

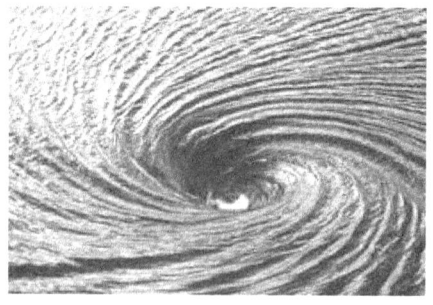

{An example of a water vortex in the Northern Hemisphere}

To draw out harmful energy from your client, reverse the spin direction visualizing the vortex as a tool for extraction. This is useful for supporting client energy systems by removing energy from tumors resulting from diseases like cancer.

Connecting with your client

The single most powerful connection between you and your client will stem from one thing. Empathy.

Although it is mechanically possible to deliver a successful Reiki treatment without Empathy, it is often surprising how significant a difference Empathy for your client will make.

Empathy is a one of the most powerful and useful emotions that you can experience when delivering a Reiki treatment. The biggest benefit of true Empathy is that it creates a very powerful emotional bond between you and the client without requiring attachment to the client. You can deliver especially powerful treatments without personally investing yourself in the treatment.

Imbue your treatment with Empathy and be astounded by the results.

When you perform a treatment

The fascinating thing about healing is that the only true healer is self. No healer actually heals, they simply assist the body to enact it's own healing processes. A doctor cannot make a bone grow. A doctor can however position bones so when the body grows them back together, they are grown back in proper alignment.

This is equally true when performing a Reiki treatment. When you are treating a client you are not actually healing the client. You are however providing the client's body with the energetic support to heal itself. This is achieved using your abilities to provide and replenish energy, which will help the body restore itself.

Your treatments may increase the speed at which the body heals itself, but still not you.

Repetition of treatments over long periods of time may prove necessary to affectively assist a client. Imbalances may re-occur after treatments are completed especially if root causes of imbalances are not fully addressed.

These root caused could be physical, emotional or even spiritual in nature.

Chapter 6: Energy Flooding With Reiki

By Ashwita Goel

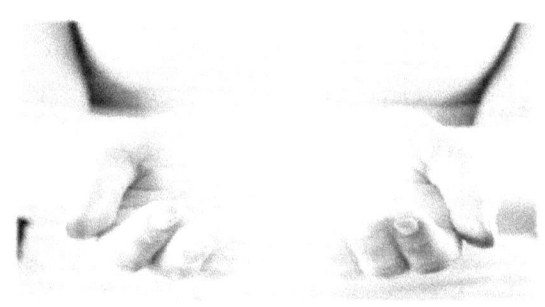

This is a really effective and quick method for flooding people and situations with energy when we feel the need for a sudden energy boost. We might want to use it if we feel that a situation might go out of hand, of if we're interacting with someone who is either angry or upset with us, or just sucking out our energy.

The Method

Imagine Reiki pour into the top of your head, filling up your whole body with energy. Once your body is full, imagine that it starts to radiate the excess energy outwards, towards the person(s) in front of you, the whole room, or the situation.

The Idea

Life throws us many situations that might find us on the backfoot. No matter what the situation, problems either begin or worsen if we give in to the reactions coming up within us. Flooding not only clears out our energy system, it also clears out the energy of the people in question, thereby creating a space for a calm and peaceful resolution.

Where we can use it

Here are some examples where flooding can be very useful:

If you find yourself trying to reason with a person who is swept away by emotion (eg. angry, hysterical or being unreasonable), this method can be quite helpful.

When you have to meet someone(s) who dislikes you or makes you uncomfortable.

When you have to address a group of people – in classrooms, in theatres, or in meetings and conference halls.

For gatherings, parties and celebrations to go smoothly, flood the entire room with pink and green energies before the event, and then continue flooding the room at periodic intervals until it is over.

While watching the news – when we feel agitated about the actions of people we haven't met, that is a very good time to practice some flooding. Not only will it clear out any negativity you might have picked up but who knows, it might bring about some healing and some change in the person the news is about.

Bear in Mind

Using this technique is not about controlling someone. If that is the primary intention behind the flooding, then it might not be effective. Remember that we are first cleansing ourselves, so let that wash away any apprehensions we might have first, and then flood the other person to turn the situation into a win-win for both. You could even mentally request the energy to do whatever is in the highest good for all the parties involved.

Creating a Reiki Altar

By Ananya Sen

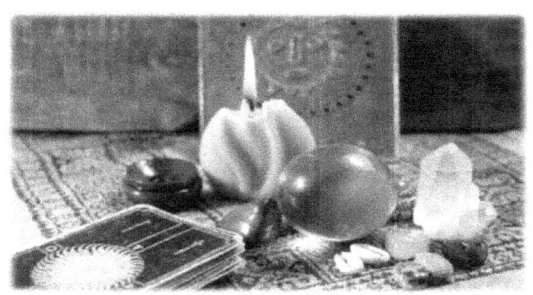

I have seen an increase in the energy flow when I channel Reiki from my altar than other parts of my home. I have also sensed an increased energy flow while sending Reiki outdoors. It is a good practice to do your daily healings and meditations from one place in your home.

When you keep praying or healing at the same spot, this becomes your meditation ground or your energy circle. This sacred space knows your personal energy so well that, it calls upon your guides the moment you step into this energy circle. I have noticed whenever I light an incense at my altar I can immediately sense the presence of some Angel or Archangel. I have been doing this for so long, that they know it's time for me to meditate or do some healing, so they immediately come by my side.

How do you create an altar? What can you keep in this altar? How do you clean your altar? First, you need to find a flat and broad surface few feet above the ground. This could be outdoor or indoor. I am of course talking about an indoor altar. You can place some Reiki or Angel photos or statues in this place. If the surface is made of marble or granite, you can just use it directly, as it will provide natural grounding when you do your energy work.

If it is wood or plastic, you can use a nice table cloth. Keep your statues on the altar. Keep your Reiki / God box on the altar. You can also place Reiki symbols on the wall near the altar or in a photo stand. I have made a large collage of all the Reiki symbols. Chakra positions and Kanji alphabets in the wall near my altar. I also have photos of Dr Mikao Usui as I really like connecting with him often.

Keep your tarot or oracle cards on the altar. Always keep a little bottle of perfume to spray on the altar. Incense and / or candles are a must, as fire cleanses negativity and clears space. Basically, keep all your healing tools in one place. They will pick up energies from each other, which is good because we tend to use one tool more than the other. This way your energy will spread evenly on your cards , statues, symbols, paintings etc. And whenever you feel a drop in your energy, you can draw energy from these charged objects.

Use rock salt and water to clean and wipe the altar. You can also run some incense or sage over the altar, because the altar also has an aura. Some practitioners keep saying their energy flow has reduced or they feel their energies are scattered, this could be one of the reasons. When you're at home channel energy from one place, you will start conserving it and your healing ability, meditation skills, mind control, visualization skills will all enhance. Create your Reiki altar today!

10 Ways to Practice Self-Care for Healing Practitioners

By Luzia Light

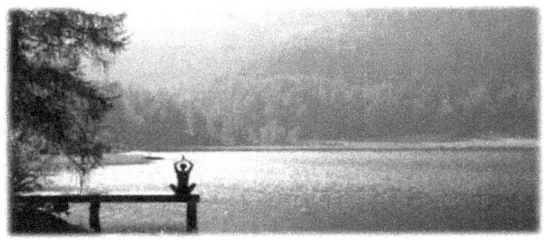

Make Self-Care a priority in your life. Many people feel guilty about making time for themselves, but when you're stressed and exhausted, you have less energy to give to others. When you begin to make self-care practices a priority in your day-to-day life, you will find that you have much more energy and patience to care for your clients. Self-care is something that you need to decide to do, because no one else will do it for you. That is true for every person, but especially for those who assist in healing and helping others.

Also, tell your clients about the importance of self-care in their own lives. In addition to helping your clients and their bodies to heal themselves, it's also important to teach them about the self-care practices they should schedule into their day. Self-care is a preventative method of healing as well as a healing method in itself. The more someone takes care of themselves with love and compassion, the easier it is for them to release the pain, struggle and resistance that made them sick in the first place.

Write yourself a list of activities that spell self-care for you! It's very personal and different for everybody. But here are some suggestions you might want to incorporate in your list:

1. **Reiki yourself daily**. At least 10-20 minutes.

2. **Meditate every morning.** 10-20 minutes. The nice thing is that you can combine the meditation with your own Reiki treatment. That can be very time efficient. :-)

3. **Exercise regularly**. That can be as simple as going for a walk in the park or taking the stairs instead of the elevator. But it's important to move your own physical energy to release the stress and tension you may have picked up from your Reiki sessions.

4. **Cut your cords**. After every treatment you give, make sure to wash your hands with cold water or cut your energy cords to the client, to make sure the energy stops flowing from you. Cutting cords can

be as simple as pretending that your right arm is a sword and moving it from top to bottom in front of your body. It's your intention that cuts the energy. You could do this in your mind as well.

5. Put your worries into a little box. Before you give a Reiki session, make sure that you are in a positive state of mind. You could visualize in your mind a little treasure box in which you put all of your own worries, stresses, irritations or arguments you may have had. Tell yourself that you can take them out of the box when you have completed the session.

6. Keep your sense of humour. Laughter can instantly shift your vibration as well as your client's. If you make little jokes, you can lighten the atmosphere and make the client feel more at ease. I find first time clients are often quite tense and anxious when they lie down on the table. I say things like: You are allowed to breathe! It's okay! :-) That at least puts a smile on their face. Remind your clients that their body can heal itself and they are the ones who own the power. You are not healing them, but you assist their bodies in healing themselves. You are just there to help.

7. Pamper yourself throughout the week. **Here are some suggestions:**

Make yourself a big cup of herbal tea and sit down in a quiet place and read a book or a magazine. If your home is not quiet, go to neighbourhood cafe.

Journal and write out all of your worries. Do a brain dump and let everything flow out. Or write your list of grievances on a piece of paper, tear it up afterwards and throw it in the garbage can where it belongs.

Go to a museum or art gallery for the afternoon.

Visit a bookstore or a library and ask your spirit guides to lead you to the book you most need to read right now.

Take your journal and write on top of the page: Dear God (Higher Self, Spirit Guide, Universe, etc.), what do I need to know right now? Then start writing without thinking and see what comes up. This can be extremely insightful. I do this almost every morning. It comforts and centers me right away.

As you go about your day, always check in with your intuition or Higher Self. Help your Higher Consciousness to make everyday decisions. Like, which way is the best route to drive home right now? What's good to make for dinner? What's the best way to spend my morning today? Who could help me with this particular challenge I have? etc.

8. Forgive yourself. Give yourself a break. Be gentle and compassionate with yourself. Forgive yourself for all the mistakes you have made in the past, and know that you are human, and humans make mistakes, it's part of the "job description". How else would we know what not to do? :-)

9. Say no to everything that doesn't nourish your soul. Never say yes just out of obligation even though inside you are squirming and screaming. Listen to your inner wisdom when you make commitments regarding your time and energy. It's perfectly okay to say: 'No, I'm not interested.' 'No, I have other priorities right now.' 'No, but I know someone you could contact who would love to help you.' etc.

10. Surround yourself with kind people. Respect yourself enough to walk away from friends who don't treat you with the love and respect you deserve. Friendships should be mutually nurturing and supportive. Hang out with people who re-energize you and love you just as you are.

Chapter 7: The Third Chakra

The third chakra is also known as the fire chakra or, in Sanskrit, the *manipura.* It deals with power and ego, and is most often the dominant chakra in an individual with imbalanced chakras. The fire chakra is located at the solar plexus. This is why, when you feel nervous, scared, and angry or loved, you might describe the experience as having butterflies or a heaviness near, and sometimes just below your solar plexus. The fire chakra is blocked by the emotion of shame.

The third chakra also governs our ability to make intimate connections with people and places we deem important. For example, the feeling of relief and happiness when you finally arrive home after being away for so long is balanced by the fire chakra. Surprisingly, the third chakra is in charge of balancing power and ego, as much as it affects the way we perceive and act in our relationships. Remember the term "power partner"? There is a reason why it is often related to intimate relationships and the existence of power struggles between the partners involved.

Opening the fire chakra

The fire chakra is important because, after learning to let go of guilt and fear, you must learn that you have the power to achieve what you want to, and be who you want to. The fire chakra teaches all individuals that true power lies in knowing how to use authority and influence to further interests, help others, and make a difference in the world. To open your third chakra, follow the simple steps detailed below.

Step 1: Look for a place where you have direct access to warmth. Preferably choose a spot that is quiet and sunny. You can also opt to sit in front of a fireplace.

Step 2: Prepare your body and mind for the experience of opening the third chakra. Recall how it felt to connect to the first and second chakras. Call upon the energy from the earth, and the water in the ground or in the air around you. Remember that all the elements, like all of your chakras are interconnected.

Step 3: Sit or stand comfortably in front of the fireplace or under the sunlight. Some people even lie down on the floor or ground just to feel the full impact of the heat on their bodies. Place your hands on your solar plexus, and breathe evenly.

Step 4: Meditate on the things, people, places and events that have made you feel powerful. Think about what you did with power and influence when you had them, and about you got them in the first place.

Step 5: Now think about the things you have done in shame. Think about how you felt. Did you feel powerless? Did you feel helpless? Did you feel like giving up? Were you ever ashamed of your weaknesses?

Step 6: Keep in mind that the third chakra teaches individuals to balance power, to use it for the good, and to help the self and others grow. Think about the times you had power and influence, how they affected your relationships and perceptions. Think about the times you were shamed and felt ashamed of yourself or your situation. Think about all these things, and slowly let them go. Imagine the powerful fire chakra consuming your shame and disappointments. Imagine the fire chakra fueling your compassion and your success.

Step 7: Breathe deeply and slowly. Every time you inhale, think about your failures. Every time you exhale, tell yourself that everyone has their own set of faults, and that, despite your shame and weaknesses; you must learn to love yourself for who you are. Realize that it is only by loving your entire identity that you grow in true, balanced power.

The fire chakra can also be strengthened by wearing or connecting with objects that have the color yellow. The third chakra can be recharged by eating foods such as pasta, cereal, bread, flax seeds, and yogurt.

Chapter 8: Reiki Self-Treatment

One of the most wonderful aspects of Reiki is the powerful ability for self-treatment and healing. Reiki self-treatment is a powerful practice. When you are ill, you can use self-treatment to speed healing. When you are well, you can use self-treatment to stay well, strengthen your health, and reduce daily stress. It is an effective immune-booster and stress buster. As Dr. Usui said, practicing self-treatment every day will keep you healthy and happy.

Mrs. Takata, the Reiki Master who brought Reiki to the West, admonished her students that self-treatment was the most important part of Reiki. First heal and treat yourself, then you can heal others. Self-care is vitally important. Recall the phrase "Love your neighbor as yourself". This phrase implies that you love yourself. You can show self-love through Reiki self-treatments and healing.

This chapter will guide you step-by-step through the self-treatment process. There are a number of differences regarding hand positions for treatment and self-treatment. Mrs. Takata had four basic positions on the front of the body and three basic positions on the back. William Lee Rand, a well-known Reiki Master, includes in his Reiki manual, 15 positions for self-treatment and 18 positions for treating others.

This book details one of many different hand position placements. Let your intuition guide you and know that Reiki can flow where it is needed. Giving self-treatment doesn't need to be complicated, merely open yourself up to Reiki and the willingness to heal.

Chapter 9: Meditation

What is meditation? Meditation is a practice whereby we focus our mind inward with the aim to discipline it and quiet it. In our modern age and time, everything is aimed at distracting us. It seems we can't even seem to drive without listening to music or the radio. There are constant distractions from us and our feelings. And in effect, when we have strong feelings or feelings that make us feel bad, all we aim to do is distract ourselves from them. This cuts us off from our inner life.

Why is it important to meditate when one does reiki? It is important when one does a reiki treatment to be able to keep our minds focused on what we do and to allow enough inner silence so that we can connect to the feelings of peace, unconditional love and detachment that are the basis to allow reiki energy to flow freely. And this cannot be done without practising meditation. It takes time and practice to be able to reach that state.

Pay attention to how many thoughts you have in one minute? If you really listen to those thoughts, you will start feeling dizzy. Your mind seems to be a constant critic and commentator of everything you do. It is actually a known fact that in teaching, things need to be repeated eleven times before they sink in, because the mind keeps on side tracking during a teaching session. There is nothing wrong with it. It just is human nature. But when you recognise this, then you understand how important it is that you train your mind. I like to compare the mind to a young stallion. It is beautiful and powerful and full of energy, but lacking any training it can become destructive and ruin your life. The mind needs constant discipline and a firm hand. It needs to understand that you are the boss. Who are you? Your soul is your essence. Many people mistake the mind for the soul. It is entirely different. The soul is so much bigger and wiser than the mind. And what you want when you do reiki is to connect to your soul.

Meditation will help you manage distractions whilst you do reiki: Distractions from the outside world; Distraction from your patient's interjections; but also as importantly, distractions from your own mind. Your own mind will nag you about the fact that you don't feel anything in your hands when you give reiki, when others brag about seeing colours and experiencing heat or cold or tingling. It will tell you that nothing is happening. Your mind will continue to haunt you by comparing you to other reiki practitioners that can see auras and tell you that unless you can do the same, what you do is pointless. Your mind will put the focus on the importance of seeing the aura and getting messages. But in reality, the mind is only the part of you that is trying to sabotage the good work that you are doing. All that matters when you do reiki is that you focus on your own inner sanctuary and find inside the overwhelming divine love that you feel for the person who comes to you. There should be no attachment to results. No attachment to what the patient feels, or does not feel. There should only be a peaceful and quiet presence. No questioning of how it went. Just gratefulness that you could be of service. Being a healer is purely being of service of what is needed for the highest good of the person that comes to you. That person may still need to continue to be ill, but you will facilitate a deep understanding of what they need to change to get better. It could be their attitude, or breaking free from an abusive relationship, or following their dreams.

Sometimes people also struggle if they have someone come to them and they seem to get worse, or at least not improve. You have to give up trying to understand what is best for the person's highest good. Even if that person died, that might be for their highest good. It might be their time to go. Who are you to think that you are here to save everyone? I know this sounds extreme, but personally I see my role to alleviate suffering and if I can hold someone's hand on their death bed and bring them peace whilst they go back to the creator, then I consider my role as a healer as complete. I have met people who think the opposite and consider that the clients who "die" on them, are personal failures. To me this says that the healer has an agenda and brings the ego to the table because they want results and to be recognised for their "powers" by the community. That is certainly not an attitude that I commend. Reiki should always be offered with no agenda and no strings attached. In fact, one should be strong enough to understand and be happy when people refuse reiki and help. If we get offended, we should see that our ego has come into the equation.

Without meditation, it is very hard to come to that state of mind and to keep it for the duration of a treatment. Meditation will bring you closer to detachment and peaceful mindfulness.

How to meditate is the next question. There are many ways to meditate. For the novice, the easier way is probably to listen to a guided meditation, either in classes or with a CD. But you must consider that meditation can be weaved into your daily life without disrupting it too much. We cannot all lead the life of a monk and sit in silence for hours on end. Consider this: meditation can be doing your ironing in silence with feelings of peace and contentment in the present moment. Meditation can be done whilst cycling. It is not so much what you do but the state of mind when you do it. It is a contemplative practice however, so I doubt you can meditate whilst doing aerobics. Maybe you can prove me wrong.

Chapter 10: How Does Angelic Reiki Energy Work

Synopsis

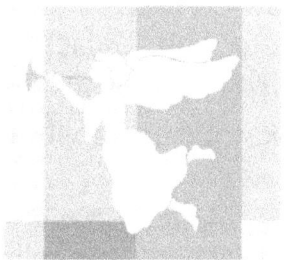

Angelic Reiki is a safe, natural, high frequency, multidimensional scheme of healing and consciousness enlargement. It's among the most potent systems of healing available at this time, yet easy to learn and simple to use.

How Does It Work

Angelic Reiki works at a Soul level, addressing the cause of any condition, advancing really deep healing and transformation. During a treatment, both practician and receiver are connected to pure divine power through the Angelic Kingdom of Light. This lets very high vibrational energies of Angels, Archangels, Ascended Masters and Galactic Healers work to help free physical, ancestral, emotional and karmic instabilities across all time.

Applying and teaching Angelic Reiki, consequently, calls for working hand-in-hand with the Angels in an unparalleled, joyful way.

There are no familiar contra-indications or areas of caution. Angelic Reiki is, consequently, suitable for anybody, of any age, and any condition may benefit from treatments. Men, women, youngsters, babies, pregnant ladies and animals may safely get Angelic Reiki alongside conventional health care and any additional complemental therapy. As the case studies illustrate, advantages are many and wide-ranging.

Angelic Reiki heals deep core issues, liberating and empowering in an unequalled way.

There's no recommended number of treatments for any condition as the treatments are client-, not practitioner-led, and clients often report favorable change after merely one treatment. But, with the exception of chronic disorders, and pregnant women who decide to have treatments throughout their pregnancy, however a treatment plan rarely involves more than 3 sessions.

During Angelic Reiki treatments the procedure of attuning to, and working with, beings of light on the higher dimensions, may supply the practitioner and the guest with insights into causes of conditions.

Treatments are carried on in a calm, safe and supportive environment and commonly last about 60 minutes. Healing frequently begins well before the practitioner and guest are face-to-face in the therapy room.

A medical and life-style history is taken during the inaugural consultation. Ample time is permitted at the beginning of every treatment for the client to talk about, if they wish, whatever is bothering them. They then sit or lie down, fully-clothed, and are asked to relax.

The practitioner produces a healing vortex and lays their hands softly on the client's body. Healing energy that's perfect in its conception and transmission is accessed by the practitioner with the Angelic Kingdom of Light, and channeled to the guest from a neutral space. If healing with Angelic Reiki is incited, both the guest and practitioner receive a down pouring of

Soul energy, and divine Angelic Archetypes are anchored, causing a transformational pitch in consciousness. Angels, Archangels, Ascended Masters and/or Galactic Healers then extend to the past to heal all memories of agony. For the receiver, any old thought-forms not in-tune with the Divine Vibration get shifted and transmuted to a higher vibration. Non-harmonious physical, emotional and mental situations are relieved, advancing really deep healing and transformation which may manifest seemingly heaven-sent physical effects.

Each treatment is unique. What the guest and the practitioner might see, feel, sense… varies substantially, and might be profound beyond words to name fully. At the close of the treatment, each discusses what has been felt, and the practitioner passes on particular Angelic Guidance.

Following the treatment, healing goes on to be absorbed at the suitable physical, emotional, psychological and spiritual level(s), and full integrating of the Angelic Healing energies may take 3 weeks or more.

Absent (distant) Angelic Reiki treatments are every bit as powerful in terms of healing strength, and the process is virtually the same, except that the client isn't physically there.

Chapter 11: The Place Of The Master/Teacher.

Reiki has been described as an oral tradition and as such has had many books written about it. Now there is one more! Not only books, but pages and pages have appeared on the Internet, not to mention my web site! We all do it; we seem to have a need to get things into the written word in order to give them credibility. Again we are trying to make things permanent, to make them true. I know the argument that this stops things from being altered and changed and this is true to a point, but books are often written for a reason and with a slant. This then, can pass into history as fact. We only have to look at fundamentalist thinking to see this in action.

The written word, after all, is only one man's interpretation at the time of writing.

It has its place and I have had a love affair with books and the written word all my life, but the fact that it is written does not make it true. Just because it is on the telly or spoken by a learned expert doesn't make it any more true. Even less true if it comes from your Reiki Master!

The Oral Tradition is not about the words that are spoken at the workshop. These words hold the same problems as the written ones and a few more of their own. It is about the process of being there, of sharing, of a commitment to listen and to stand back and accept, even if it is only for a short space of time. You should come away not with answers but with questions. But you should also possess a tool that helps you find the answers to those questions. It is the doing that matters. So it is not just a matter of e-mailing Amazon and then reading the book at your convenience. You have to make that commitment to find out about Reiki, to participate (even to the degree of spending money and exchanging your energy,) then the process of attunement starts and the connection is recognised. It's the doing and being there that matters.

Often the people I have attuned to Reiki will tell me that once they had committed themselves to attending a workshop they felt different; that things started to happen almost as if they had already attended. I have been told this so many times that I must start to accept it. Certainly I know that once I have committed myself to holding a workshop people come. I can't ``force" how many or who comes, no matter how hard I try and I now know that, without exception, the groups gel. Sometimes better than others, but, unlikely as it seems and as different as they might be, they get along. I used to worry when I looked at the group of people destined for the next weekend. I would try to get a good mix of like-minded people but it never worked out the way I planned. The workshops just sorted themselves out and the right people, for that workshop, booked and came, despite me, despite my efforts. Now I don't try, I just set out my stall and trust.

The Reiki Master has his place too, bless his little cotton socks, not as a conveyor of great wisdom, or some sort of high priest. Remember that the only difference between you, who has just started in Reiki, and the Reiki Master, is experience. That's all! (Well, maybe he is a bloke and you're a girl, but you know what I mean.) The ability of both of you to give Reiki is the same; he has just done it before and has made the mistakes first. Don't be fooled otherwise.

So why would anyone want to be a Reiki master? Well, ego plays a part; I want the biggest and best, sort of thing. This comes from a misunderstanding of Reiki. There is no ladder to climb, no ``more powerful" givers of Reiki. Remember we don't give the Reiki, it is received. Then there is the need to confirm that what you are doing is right by getting others to join our club. (And believe me sometimes you do need a little support, especially when you start wondering if you have lost the plot). You see this attitude not only with Reiki but with all sort of things; cars, TVs, mobile phones.

"I just bought this wonderful new thing. It's the best ever! You just must get one." And so we do, and if it's good, great, and if it's not… anyone want a Betamax video or a mini disc player?

There are many reasons why people want to become Reiki Masters but firstly you should want to pass on Reiki; to teach. If you don't you are wasting your time and money. In the dim and distant past it used to cost a lot of cash and you had to be invited to become a Reiki Master. This made you think if you really wanted to commit yourself. The cost used to be one week's wage for First Degree, I month's for Second Degree and a year's for Masters. Maybe too much and I feel that it was unrealistic. But it did make you stop and think. It made you consider if you really wanted to teach. Now you can get the whole package for 50 quid all in one weekend and this has flooded the market with Reiki masters with little knowledge and only one week's experience. You get the ``what shall we do for the weekend? I know, lets become Reiki Masters brigade''. When you choose who will attune you, bare this in mind. Like a puppy at Christmas your Reiki Master is not just for your attunements, but for life (if you want). This is his/her commitment to you. The Reiki master's job is to pass on the attunements then help you avoid all the mistakes they have made and give support as and when you need it. And that's all.

An interesting thing happens between a Reiki Master and the Masters he attunes. It has a similar parallel to what happens when you first start off with Reiki. When you are first attuned to Reiki you are a little unsure and all your treatments resemble the way you learnt to give them at your workshop, blow for blow, hand position for hand position; very simple, straight forward treatments. After a bit, as your confidence grows, you start to be more adventurous and your treatments get more complicated and involved. You develop your style. More time passes, you do more treatments and you get more experience and you find that your treatments change again; once more they become very simple! It's funny but we all seem to need to go through this progression.

A similar thing happens when you become a Reiki Master. You copy your Master like a mirror and teach simply. After a while you realise that your Master did not understand the whole picture and your teaching becomes more in-depth, more meaningful. Time passes and, blow me down, you find yourself teaching simply again. Not trying to understand the whole picture, not trying to show others what it is all about, but just doing and letting others find out for themselves the beauty of simplicity. We all do this and it seems necessary, so don't worry when you find yourself thinking, that nutty old guy didn't know what he was talking about. He probably didn't, but what was passed on to you was more important than words and you will sort it out for yourself and in the way that best suits you. So pat him on the head and humour him. He's harmless!

The attunements are the keys with which we bring our body's energetic system back into harmony with the rest of creation - and that's creation with a capital C. Once back and recognised, we can start to re-balance the whole body. Best of all we start to remember what that balance feels like and store that memory away like an old tuning fork. Then, when we find ourselves going out of tune, we can dig around in our ``sock draw", dust off our life's tuning fork, give it a good bang and remember how life should sound. The attunements set our personal tuning forks back to resonate with the universal one. The Reiki Master does the banging and we hum along.

For a Reiki Master, giving the attunements is a very special thing and a great privilege. Every time is different and unique. I have often wondered if the physical act of giving an attunement is needed or if the attunement happens when the commitment takes place. I don't know. Anyway, the process of the attunements is nice and, as I said before, rather special. It is the pivot point of my workshops and seems to unite people. It is funny, but the difference in a group before and after that first attunement is measurable; slightly reserved before, chatting away and laughing together after. So if it works, don't mend it!

Chapter 12: How To Perform Reiki

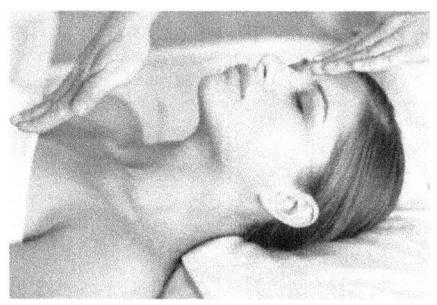

Reiki is very simple, and someone who is interested can easily learn it and perform it as self-heal. Adults, elderly or children ... anyone can learn this practice. You do not need to have a special set of skills or a significant educational background to receive training. One of the best things about Reiki is that it will only take about 10 hours for you to learn it.

Receiving Reiki treatment from someone else is wonderful, but it can be really advantageous to learn it yourself. Not only is it convenient but you easily perform it on yourself whenever and wherever you need it. Despite your busy schedule, you will always find the time to relax if you know how to perform Reiki.

If you perform Reiki daily, you will be able to restore your body's balance, reduce tension and stress, improve your overall wellness, relieve discomfort and pain and ease anxiety. Both the healthy and those with health conditions can benefit from Reiki. They can perform it every day to relieve pain or to simply strengthen their bodies.

How can you learn Reiki?

The only way to learn Reiki is by having a qualified Reiki master teach you. Of course, you will need to find a Reiki master and you can do that by searching groups or friends who practice Reiki. You can also inquire with masseuses or therapists, as they usually know therapy providers. You can also check yoga centers, search online, hospitals and even health stores to find out if they know anyone. Reiki is widely used and received by many people who suffer from certain conditions, thus, it will also make sense to check organizations that cater to people with illnesses and ask if they have a list of Reiki masters.

While you are searching for a Reiki master, always keep in mind that it is not a standardized or regulated practice so there is no guarantee that a person calling himself a Reiki master has completed training and has enough experience. Due to this reason, it is very important that you ask the Reiki master specific questions. If he or she is truly a Reiki master, he or she should have no problem answering your questions.

A lot of Reiki masters and practitioners advertise through websites, leaflets or brochures. It is there where they describe their experiences, their training and their methods of teaching. If you feel like the information on there is not enough, set aside some time to meet with the Reiki master and have a brief discussion with him or her to make sure that he or she meets what you are looking for in a teacher. Ask about the way he or she teaches his or her classes—the schedule and his or her fee, as well as the opportunities that he or she can offer with regard to continued mentoring. Take your time in looking for a Reiki master. You need to be careful with who you choose, as he or she should not be a teacher that not only has the qualifications, but someone who you are also comfortable with.

Here are some of the basic hand positions that you can do when you perform Reiki on yourself:

Place your hands on top of your head, and make sure one hand is on top of the other.

Place one hand on your forehead and place the other on the back of your head in between the crown of your head and the base of your skull.

Gently rest your hands on your eyes.

Gently rest your hands on your ears.

Place one hand on your upper chest and the other on the place where your ribs meet.

Lightly place your hands on your hips.

Every time you position your hands, relax them there for 2 to 5 minutes. Keep on practicing these hand positions until you become familiar and comfortable with them. Over time, you will learn to let your hands be guided with your intuition.

What are the three degrees of Reiki training?

Reiki training consists of 3 degrees which build on top of the other. Each has a different goal and scope of practice, although the laying on of hands still remains the foundation of all degrees.

First degree. The first degree usually takes 8 to 12 hours to be taught. Students are taught how to self-treat and perform Reiki on one another. It is in this degree wherein the students are prepared to perform Reiki on themselves daily. They are taught the correct hand placements, as well as how to place them when performing on family and friends. Some may be executed in one full session or in a chair session. They are also taught how to treat when in dire situations and how to perform on the spot.

Reiki courses are offered to health care professionals like nurses and caregivers.

Often, their courses include the application of Reiki in clinical settings. During this time, the Reiki master discusses the history and the concepts of Reiki. The Reiki master also initiates the students for them to become effective mediums of Reiki energy. First-degree training usually involves four initiation levels that only a Reiki master can fully discuss. If you only wish to self-heal and perform on family and friends, first-degree training is all you need.

Second degree. Second degree is also called distant healing. Now, students are taught how to replace the contact between the hand and the body with a mental connection, so that they can still perform Reiki and continue to heal even if a physical connection is inappropriate or is physically impossible. If there is still physical contact, second-degree or distant healing can be used to further enhance the first degree, which is the hands-on treatment.

Third degree. The third degree depends on the Reiki master. Before, it was tradition for the Reiki master to invite or to train only those people whom he or she thought were fully prepared to dedicate their lives to teaching the practice to others. Third-degree training or master training is taught not through lectures, practical examples or course work, but through a comprehensive and lengthy apprenticeship with the Reiki master. Remember, only a real Reiki master can effectively teach Reiki to others.

The only way to successfully learn Reiki, aside from being taught by a Reiki master, is to practice. You can self-treat yourself daily or perform on your family and friends to improve their overall well-being or to improve health conditions and illnesses. Consistent practice of Reiki can engage the people participating in a culture which embraces wellness, gives importance to bonding, exudes positivity and creates habits of healthy living that can support a lifetime of health and happiness.

Chapter 13: The Practice Of Reiki

Western, conventional medicine differs in a lot of ways to Reiki as it involves diagnosing and applying specific drugs and treatments to combat ills in the body. Reiki rather charts a tunnel through which healing energy permeates the patient through the practitioner. The receiver receives it directly from the practitioner through specific hand positions each communicating a definite purpose. For the energy to thoroughly permeate, direct contact isn't a requirement.

Reiki Levels

Reiki has three substantiate standard levels and the first and most basic of them opens you up to the sway of your Reiki healing energy channels. You are not ordinary again even at this level for you have mastered a major skill in life in the ability to wield the energy of the universe to heal yourself and others. Different Reiki levels correspond to varying amount of healing energy that you can channel. Level III is that of a master and the energy you can wield there is greater than II and I. A level I practitioner is operating at the basic level and a level II practitioner is more opened to additional healing methods which include the procedure of symbols and distant healing. Some unique set of Reiki practitioners who have become masters can teach others from level I to III.

Healing Others

After the process of attunement and you are confirmed a level I degree Reiki practitioner, you can start off by healing other people. There are many ways you can go about it when about to give hands-on healing which includes asking them to lie down—which is the most convenient for both because the practitioner gets all the comfort in this world and access to all chakras— or sit. Lying down also ensures that the patient feels a lot more relaxed for the unfolding Reiki session. A loose-fitting, comfortable clothing is the best for the patient and you should advise that if you had the chance to talk with them in advance.

Apart from gold and silver jewelry which may be worn, as soon as before they touch the table or chair, request for the removal of others like a watch, jewelry, spectacles, belt and etc. Both of you could do with a glass of water as it relaxes you both and keeps you in alignment. Ensure that they lay comfortably, often on their back with eyes closed, and starts the healing procedure from their brow chakra through all the front chakras. From there you move into all other aspects of the session in correspondence to the result you are both working at.

Distance Healing

As a Reiki I practitioner you need some level of contact with the patient but it is in Level II that you really begin to grasp and deploy the way of the universal energy. Mastering Reiki to level II means you can send this energy anywhere and to anyone as you have successfully opened the channels that are only attuned to level II and above. Sending energy to someone distant requires a specific set of considerations to enhance the level of effectiveness. First, time must be set apart by them so as to adequately receive the Reiki energy sent to them with all good intentions. That ensures that the healing energy that reaches them is received with a raised consciousness which directly impacts their chance at healing their own bodies.

Let them sit, close their eyes and keep their feet on the floor without having their hands or leg crossed over. Let them at least try to heighten their awareness and feel the energy emanating towards them. Distant energy can be sent through several ways: from using a photograph of the recipient; to using an object as a surrogate; to making use of an intention slip; or having them vivid in the imagination, or simply release Reiki to them through the third eye.

Chapter 14: Solving Problems The Reiki Way

Synopsis

Almost everyone who has had some encounters with the reiki world of positive energy practices sings its praises. Touted to be a beautiful and calming practice, many believe it is one art form the world at large can benefit from being exposed to it.

The Benefits

Most diseases, mind conditions and even the abuse of the environment has been linked to the negative elements at one time or another. The practice of reiki, can to some extent eliminate this negative aspect or energy, and replace it with positive energy.

Reiki's positive energy addresses the mind, body, and surroundings that connect it altogether one way or another. When reiki is used to address the mind, elements like the thought process, can be tuned to only consist of positive thoughts.

When the state of mind is trained to always be positive, a lot of good can be achieved and even transcend into the surroundings. Besides the thought process, the reiki style of transferring positive energy unto another can help create a better state of actual mental health. Headaches, migraines, stress, and other brain related problems can be successfully addressed with the positive energy of reiki.

Considered to be relatively "free", reiki art of transferring positive energy also works when applied to address ailments in the body. This positive reiki energy is used to flush out any negative energy which may be contributing to the ill health of the individual.

Reiki's positive energy transfer does not involve any amount of pain or discomfort. In fact most people have attested to experiencing a comforting warm feeling which in some cases causes such relaxation that dozing off during a session is not unusual.

Reiki has also been known for its distance healing abilities. This unusual feature is another advantage to those seeking this type of healing to compliment an ongoing medicinal regiment. An experienced reiki practitioner can transfer positive energy through quiet meditation quite successfully.

Chapter 15: Human Physiology

The human body is a miraculous machine. It performs many complex functions, each of which helps us live. The body is made up of billions of microscopic cells, each contributing to keeping the body functioning and growing. Collections of similar cells form tissues. A collection of similar tissues acting together to perform a specific function are called organs. A group of organs and other structures specially adapted to perform specific body functions are called a body system.

There are five primary body systems we will study in Level 1. This chapter covers each system briefly. It is recommended you develop a deeper understanding of these systems and other aspects of human anatomy as you grow as a Reiki practitioner.

ENDOCRINE SYSTEM

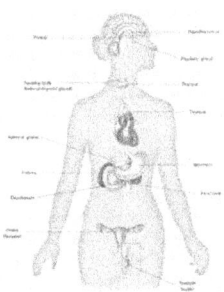

The endocrine system secretes hormones and other substances into the blood and onto the skin.

Thyroid Gland

 Located in the front of the neck. Secretes thyroid hormone.
 Regulates the body's overall metabolism.

Parathyroid Glands

⊞ Consists of four glands located behind the thyroid. Secretes parathyroid hormone.
⊞ Has absolute control over calcium levels throughout the body.

Adrenal Glands

⊞ Consists of two glands located on the top of each kidney. The inner part secretes adrenaline; the outer secretes aldosterone and cortisol.

⊞ Maintains salt levels in the blood, maintains blood pressure, helps control kidney function, and controls overall fluid concentrations in the body.

Neuroendocrine Glands (Pancreas)

⊞ Located deep in the abdomen behind the stomach, the pancreas is primarily a digestive organ.
⊞ Contains extremely important endocrine cells, which secrete insulin,

glucagon, somatostatin, and others.

- Controls blood sugar and overall glucose metabolism, and helps control other endocrine cells of the digestive tract.

Pituitary Gland

- Located at the base of the brain.

- Secretes thyroid stimulating hormone (TSH), follicle stimulating hormone (FSH), adrenocotropic hormone (ACTH), and others.

- Controls the activity of many other endocrine glands (thyroid, ovaries, adrenal, etc.).

DIGESTIVE SYSTEM

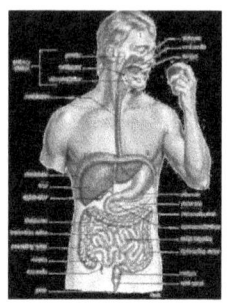

The digestive system breaks down food into usable forms to supply the rest of the body with energy.

Mouth

⊡ Located at the front of the face where speech takes place.

⊡ Food is partly broken down by the process of chewing (with the teeth and tongue) and by the chemical action of enzymes from the salivary glands that break down starches into smaller molecules.

Esophagus

📖 A long tube that runs from the mouth to the stomach.

📖 It uses rhythmic, wavelike muscle movements (called peristalsis) to force food from the throat into the stomach.

Stomach

📖 A hollow, saclike organ connected to the esophagus and the small intestine.

📖 Both chemical and mechanical digestion takes place in the stomach. When food enters the stomach, it is churned in a bath of acids and enzymes.

📖 The stomach serves as: (1) a storage bin, holding a meal in the upper portion and releasing it a little at a time into the lower portion for processing; (2) a food mixer, the strong muscles contract and mash the food into a sticky, slushy mass; (3) a sterilizing system, where the cells in the stomach produce an acid which kills germs in "bad" food; (4) a digestive tub, the stomach produces digestive fluid which splits and cracks the chemicals in food to be distributed as fuel for the body.

Small Intestine

▫ A long, continuous tube running from the stomach to the large intestines, about 20 feet long and about an inch in diameter.

▫ Breaks down most sugars and proteins and absorbs monosaccharides, amino acids, as well as water and electrolytes.

▫ Also acts as a barrier by separating the lumen of the digestive tract.

Large Intestine/Colon

▫ Located in the abdominal cavity. The first part is called the cecum and it is in the lowerright quadrant, just inside the hip bone.

▫ The next apt, the ascending colon,

goes up at an angle up to about the tenth rib.

▢ Then, the transverse colon goes across the front of the abdomen under the ribs and above the navel to the left side—about the tenth rib.

▢ Then, it goes down to just inside the other hip bone and becomes the descending colon.

▢ The next part is called the sigmoid colon and it makes an S-shape that goes deeper into the abdomen and becomes the rectum.

▢ The last part is an opening called the anus. The colon absorbs fluids and recycles them into the blood stream.

▢ The second half compacts the wastes into feces, secretes mucus which binds the substances, and lubricates it to protect the colon and ease its passage.

Pancreas

 An enzyme-producing gland located below the stomach and above the intestines.

 Enzymes from the pancreas help in the digestion of carbohydrates, fats and proteins in the small intestine.

Gallbladder

 A small, sac-like organ located by the duodenum.

 It stores and releases bile (a digestive chemical produced in the liver) into the small intestine.

Liver

 A large organ located above and in front of the stomach. It filters toxins from the blood, and makes bile (which breaks down fats) and some blood proteins.

RESPIRATORY SYSTEM

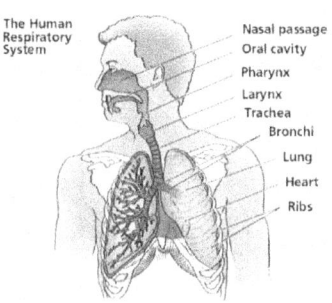

The respiratory system supplies the blood with oxygen in order for the blood to deliver oxygen to all parts of the body. The respiratory system does this through breathing. When we breathe, we inhale oxygen and exhale carbon dioxide. This exchange of gases is the respiratory system's means of getting oxygen to the blood.

Mouth and Nose

Oxygen enters the respiratory system through these. The nose filters dust and other disease-causing agents out of the air and into the body and releases exhaled air.

Trachea

☐☐ A tube that enters the chest cavity that transports air from mouth and nose into the chest, upon exhalation just the opposite direction

Bronchi

☐☐ Small tubes that lead directly into the lung tissue that distribute air to and from the lungs.

Alveoli

☐☐ These tiny spongy sacs in the lungs surrounded by capillaries diffuse oxygen into the surrounding arterial blood, diffusing carbon dioxide out from the veinous blood.

Diaphragm

◻ This is a sheet of muscles that lie across the bottom of the chest cavity.
◻ They help pump the carbon dioxide out of the lungs and pull the oxygen into the lungs.

◻ As the diaphragm contracts and relaxes, breathing takes place. When the diaphragm contracts, oxygen is pulled into the lungs. When the diaphragm relaxes, carbon dioxide is pumped out of the lungs.

CIRCULATORY SYSTEM

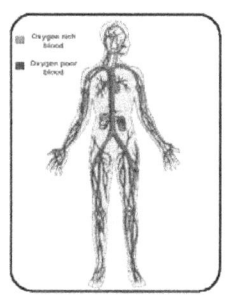

The circulatory system transports nutrients and oxygen to the body's cells and removes waste products.

Heart

 Located in the center of your chest slightly to the left.
 It pumps your blood and keeps the blood moving throughout your body.

Blood

 This substance is constantly flowing through our bodies, traveling through thousands of miles of blood vessels.
 Red blood cells carry oxygen to cells and carbon dioxide out of cells.
 White blood cells help the body fight off germs.
 Platelets stop bleeding.
 Plasma, the liquid part of the blood, is made in the liver.
 Your blood carries nutrients, water, oxygen and waste products to and from your body cells.

Blood Vessels

☐☐ These are veins, arteries and capillaries that carry blood to and from the heart and transport blood to all the cells of the body.

URINARY SYSTEM

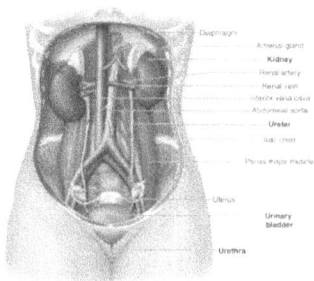

Removes waste from the circulatory system and regulates water balance.

Urinary System

☐☐ Filters waste and extra fluid from your blood.

Kidneys

▫️ These bean-shaped organs are about the size of fists. They are near the middle of the back, just below the rib cage.

▫️ They remove urea from the blood. Urea, together with water and other waste substances, forms the urine.

Ureters

▫️ Tubes about 8 to 10 inches long leading from the kidneys to the bladder.
▫️ They transport wastes from kidneys to bladder.

Bladder

▫️ A hollow, muscular organ shaped like a balloon. It sits in the pelvis and is held in place by ligaments attached to other organs and the pelvic bones.

▫️ Swells to hold urine. If the urinary system is healthy, the bladder can hold up to 16 ounces (2 cups) of urine comfortably for 2 to 5 hours.

Sphincters

▢ Circular muscles that close tightly like a rubber band around the opening of the bladder into the urethra, the tube that allows urine to pass outside the body.

▢ Nerves in the bladder tell you when it is time to empty your bladder. As the bladder fills with urine, you may notice a feeling that you need to urinate. The sensation becomes stronger as the bladder continues filling and reaches its limit. At that point, nerves from the bladder send a message to the brain that the bladder is full, and your urge to empty your bladder intensifies.

▢ When you urinate, the brain signals the bladder muscles to tighten, squeezing urine out of the bladder. At the same time, the brain signals the sphincter muscles to relax. As these muscles relax, urine exits the bladder through the urethra. When all the signals occur in the correct order, normal urination takes place.

Chapter 16: The Process Of Attunement

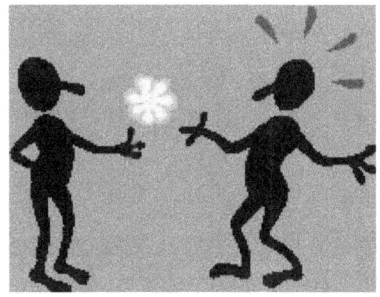

The process of attuning people to Reiki energy is at the heart of the workshop experience. By drawing the Reiki symbols into the recipient's energy field, you are introducing them to the energy flow from the circle of the Reiki Masters. As a Reiki teacher/attuner you enable others to channel the energy. Once a recipient is empowered with Reiki, they will have it for the rest of their lives.

Practise attunements on a daily basis until your ability to visualise the symbols, draw the symbols, and perform the attunements is smooth, flowing, and confident. Practice on your friends, family, and pets. Doing the attunements can be an exhilarating experience. Pace yourself and keep records of your changes.

We encourage you to practice the attunements for as long as *you* need before you begin to teach. This allows the energy to anchor and you to integrate this new capacity into your life. During this time, keep a journal of your experiences, dreams, visions, and plans. Please write to me at the end of that period and let your attuner know your experience. You are also free to call at any time to ask questions or to receive additional support.

It is up to your inner knowing when it is time to teach. Be aware of your sensations during the attunement and check the recipient's hands afterwards. Are they channelling Reiki energy? Let your guidance and integrity tell you when you have mastered the art of Reiki attunement and the responsibility of ushering people into the circle in a clear and loving manner. Then share it fully and lovingly.

Every time you do an attunement you are also attuned. Your own energy expands in the interconnectedness between you and the whole circle of Reiki Healers shines. Accept the changes with grace.

About The Attunements Generally

People learning **First** Degree Reiki receive **four** First Degree Attunements within two days. Each attunement is the same. However, each time the student receives an attunement, the Reiki energy becomes more firmly anchored in the recipient's energy body. Usually anyone who requests it get Reiki One. We always emphasise it is intended for their own use only. In First

Degree the instructions in *italics* are done *once.*

Teach the **Second** Degree **at least** three weeks after the First Degree. **Two** Second Degree Attunements are given within the space of two days or less. Teach as required dependant on the availability of time, and number of participants. Reiki Two may be used as widely as desired by the recipient. In Second Degree the instructions in *italics* are done *twice.*

Third Degree is passed when both the teacher and pupil agree it is appropriate. **Three** Third Degree Attunements are given within two days. Reiki Three can be just for own development, to pass on Heart attunements or as a step towards becoming a full teacher/attuner. Contact with the master who attuned you for a lengthy period afterwards is desirable. In the Third Degree the instructions in *italics* are done *thrice.*

If You Make a Mistake During an Attunement ...

If, for instance, you do not draw a symbol correctly, stop drawing the symbol, pump your Hui Yin *three* times, and redraw the symbol from the beginning. You do not need to start the entire sequence of symbols over, only the one you were drawing when the error occurred. As you redraw the symbol, remember to say the name silently *three* times.

Follow these steps when initiating one or more persons. If there are more than six it may be preferable to divide the group, with some taking a break whilst other are attuned. Make it clear what is expected to hold the group energies in the break times. Generally include the same elements of group process, meditation, practice, creating the circle, and accessing the healer within, in the First, Second and Third Degree Workshops.

Chapter 17: Working Honestly

The fourth Reiki principle is "Just for today do your work honestly". This one often causes confusion or misunderstanding as there are various translations for it and we have various ideas of what "work" is!

Some of the other translations are "Do your work diligently" or "Work hard".

Was Usui telling us to be slaves to the grind? I don't believe so.

What is work?

When you hear the word "work" – what springs to mind for you?

Is it your paid employment? Perhaps it is your everyday tasks or chores? Do you have a positive mental picture of "work" or is it something that fills you with dread?

In today's Western society, we are working long hours and stress is a massive problem. In the UK we have the work/life balance all out of sync! People are tending to work longer and longer hours and as a result their health is suffering.

Health & Safety Executive Statistics show that stress affects one in five of the working population from the newest recruit in the post room to the board of directors. It is now the single biggest cause of sickness in the UK. Over 105 million days are lost to stress each year – costing UK employers £1.24 billion.

So is Usui telling us that this is the way to live when he says "Just for today work hard"?

No I believe we are being told to work in a way that is in alignment with our integrity and to work hard on ourselves. I'll come back to this in a moment – let's look at the stress we face in our working lives first of all.

It is important to remember that a certain amount of stress is a good thing. It helps you perform better and spurs you on to take action when it is needed.

The main thing, with stress management, is to learn how to turn your stress to your advantage rather than let it overwhelm you.

Some people find they thrive with a little bit of stress – it pushes them forward and helps them climb to new heights. These people have a coping mechanism whereby they are able to manage their stress.

Other people don't find it so easy. They become overwhelmed and start to display the signs and symptoms of stress. They begin to sink rather than swim and this is when it is obviously a problem.

There is a stress line – those who stay above the line are less affected by stress than those who fall beneath it. Those who are visionaries, self-motivated and dynamic are said to be above the stress line while those who are stressed out, survival orientated and bureaucratic are beneath the line.

Where would you put yourself?

Your attitude is the key to this question. Do you work willingly and with a good heart or are you a reluctant worker who feels they "have to" do the work as they have no choice?

Do you value your work? How do you feel about what you do? What is your role? What drives and motivates you? What are your ambitions or dreams?

When you start to dig into these questions you begin to question your life purpose and this is what I feel Usui was getting at with this principle. Reiki sparks change — it always does.

Change is good — it helps us to grow and develop and that is really what Reiki is all about — making mindful changes towards healing our lives and living on purpose.

When Usui stated "Just for today do your work honestly" he wasn't insinuating that you are dishonest. He wasn't asking you not to steal supplies from the office or to stop using the office printer for personal use! He was asking you to be honest with yourself.

To accept yourself for who you are and for you to really know who you are.

Human Being not Human Doing

We often confuse who we are with what we do.

How many times has someone met you and asked "So what do you do then?" It seems we allow our job role to define us as a person. We must remember that we are human beings not human doings!

Usui was asking us to take a long look at ourselves and to work hard on ourselves with honesty and integrity. **You are your life's work** so you should work hard at it every day.

As you work with Reiki healing energy you may find that your 9 to 5 no longer feels right for you and is no longer in alignment with who you are. This is what happened to me.

I always got stuck with this principle. I was working in a relatively stressful IT job as a manager for a local company and the stress and pressure felt really out of alignment with who I was becoming.

I had opened up to Reiki healing energy and was on a journey of self-discovery and being stressed every day and fuelling up with coffee and red bull to get through the day simply wasn't right for me anymore.

It was more than just work though, it was my home life too.

Your work, in the context of this principle, is everything – your life, your day to day tasks, your thoughts, your personal development and your paid work. I began to take a long and honest look at my life and where it was going and I decided that changes needed to be made.

I moved from the stressful manager's job to a less stressful environment. I knew that I wouldn't stay in that job forever but it was a stepping stone for me – I began to see the bigger picture and I realised that I wanted to be my own boss and work for the good of others, not for the good of some nameless multi-national company!

I began to put plans in place for my move to self-employment. I set goals and targets for myself and I trained up and learned new skills. I began to run my business outside of normal working hours and I started to save a bit of cash to help me through the first year of self-employment.

Outside of work I also took a look at my relationships – friendships and marriage. I had to make changes and I made the decision to follow my heart and end my marriage. That wasn't easy but I knew it was right and honest for me.

It was me "doing my work honestly". I had to work hard on myself and move through the barriers and walls I had put up. I had to break down the facade of living a lie and be honest.

Often we find ourselves desperately trying to fill a void within ourselves. Something feels empty and we need to fill it so we look around externally. We accumulate more stuff and more things but that doesn't work. We perhaps turn to alcohol or other destructive behaviours and that doesn't work either.

Reiki helps us to see that the answer lies within ourselves and this is what I feel Usui was getting at.

Getting to work on yourself

Your "work" is your personal journey through life. You are a spiritual "being" having a human experience. Your journey is unique to you and Usui was asking that you work hard on yourself.

How do you work hard on yourself?

Well perhaps you may decide to start by learning Reiki for yourself – the Reiki principles and meditations certainly help you to start the process of self development and healing!

You can also read inspirational books – there are a multitude of them available nowadays. The secret is, though, to put into practice what you read and not just read about it!

Perhaps taking up a mindful or meditative practice like yoga, t'ai chi or qi gong would be helpful. I know that personally I have grown and improved since attending regular qi gong and t'ai chi classes alongside my Reiki practice.

Simply getting out in nature really helps with your personal and spiritual development too. Being in tune with nature and working with our Mother Earth really helps you connect and feel grounded in this life.

Study and learning are also important ways of developing. When was the last time you learned something new? It helps to keep the mind active and gives you new avenues to explore – there are so many free online resources out there that there is no excuse not to keep learning new things. I love it – I am a perpetual student of life!

Usui was asking us to get spiritually fit!

This requires effort and commitment in much the same way as getting physically fit does.

For physical fitness you are expected to be mindful of your diet and to carry out certain exercise regimes.

For spiritual fitness you need to live consciously and mindfully. You need to be grounded, clear and compassionate. You need to learn to see the bigger picture and find your joy.

Find your joy

The Dalai Lama is quoted as saying "The purpose of life is to be happy!"

How wonderful! That is all we want and need in life – happiness.

Usui tells us this in the principles – he calls them "The secret art of inviting happiness …"

Write down 10 things that make you happy – for example my list may be: -

Spending quality time with my partner and children.

Having time to paint and create art.

Writing and sharing my experiences.

Practising Reiki.

Travelling to new places.

Soaking up the sunshine.

Walking in nature.

Listening to music and singing (badly) at the top of my voice.

Being organised and tidy.

Laughing with my friends.

What are your 10 things? Make a note of them and then commit to integrating them into your life. By doing this you will begin to find your joy and in turn this helps you with your spiritual development.

Chapter 18: Reiki And Karma

There are so many confusions and misconceptions related to Reiki and Karma. Dr. Mikao Usui did a lot of research and meditated for years to get to know about this wonderful healing energy. He didn't just do it for his personal gain, after learning about this miraculous power he healed and taught it to many people. His main goal was to make people know their "True Self" – and achieve better health and happiness.

Hospitals cure physical and mental illness using medicines, but still there are numerous cases which couldn't be diagnosed or healed through medicine. Medical science is necessary as well as the healing science. If both go hand -in -hand the ratio of sufferings, illness and mental health will improve drastically.

Some people without knowing Reiki in depth ask not to Practice Reiki and clear Karma. For instance; when someone is in trouble (emotional, physical or mental) his intuition won't work properly. Thus he will make wrong decisions and end up in pain. When he goes through pain or suffering and take it in-depth, it will automatically convert into suffering, which will trouble him as well as his loved ones who are trying to help him get out of that situation. In this way he may add up much more Karma instead of clearing accumulated Karma.

Reiki helps to clear Karma through knowledge. This universal energy which flows through our physical body removes negative blockages and helps us to maintain peace of mind and stay calm even in tough situations. It helps us to analyze any situation or problem in broader point of view instead of complaining or getting angry. Thus, helps in reducing accumulated Karma as well as helps in creating good Agami [future] Karma.

Our physical body is surrounded by a layer called Magnetic field or Aura, which stores all the information, actions, feelings etc. Although we leave our physical body after certain time, our Magnetic field/ Aura remains the same for many lifetimes.

Any good or bad Karma which we have done at present or in the past will first reflect on our magnetic field then slowly will be transmitted to our subconscious mind. The sub-conscious mind will automatically give reward or punishment based on our thoughts. Sub-conscious mind operates on the principle of *"What you sow, you reap".* We get good for good and evil for evil. There is no injustice.

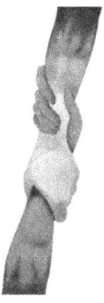

Our sub-conscious mind even without our knowledge gives us justice; our mind will not even know what is going around. Sometimes it teaches us Chapter through mental, emotional, physical pain or happiness.

Our fate is never truly set, we have free will; we can design our future through positive thoughts or deeds. We create our own reality and our own Karma through the process of thought forms, by practising Reiki daily our thought forms change positively without much effort. Reiki develops confidence, patience and helps us to cultivate gratitude towards all.

Taking responsibility of your life, practising Reiki and following the path of Dharma helps you to stay positive no matter whatever the situation is. It brings balance in your life.

Steps for self – improvement:

☐ Gain knowledge

☐ Rectify your mistakes

☐ Take action to change for better

☐ Always "Watch/observe" what you think

Chapter 19: Yoga Poses For Beginners

There are some standard yoga poses that you will be taught by teachers and it's nice to know what they mean when they say things like **downward facing dog** because without knowing what that means, you are a little at a loss. Thus, this chapter is all about standard beginner poses that you can incorporate into your workout.

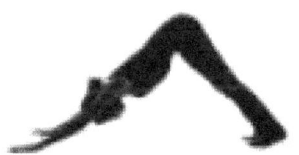

This is the downward facing dog and how this is achieved by starting on your knees on your yoga mat. If you try to achieve this in another way, you can hurt your back and that's not the purpose of the exercise.

Now, lean forward so that you are on all fours. Your thighs should be straight upward and your arms straight down so that you form a rectangle underneath your body between you and the mat. The hands should be flat with the palms against the mat and the fingers spread out. These should be directly under your shoulders. Curl your toes up so that you are leaning on the area just under your toes and then gradually pull yourself upward until your body forms an inverted V with the ground below it. Now start to press your upper body toward your legs so that your spine is straight but that V is more pronounced. Some people have difficulty and say that they can't stretch the back enough, and in order to do this, there is a little cheat, which is acceptable. Bend your knees just a little bit and then stretch your back, straightening the knees as you do this.

The next exercise is also a classic one and it is called the **Mountain Pose** for a very good reason. You think of mountains as being high places and this is about as high as you can get with a yoga movement.

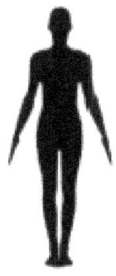

Start by standing in this position, feet flat on the mat, arms out by your side and start to breathe in and out, making yourself ready for the movement of your body. Breathe in – Exhale and move the arms upward to the sky and at the same time stand on your toes so that you are stretched as high as you possibly can be toward the sky. Hold that moment.

Breathe in and out and then swan dive the arms back down to your sides and flatten your feet against the mat. The reason that this exercise is particularly good for new yoga practitioners is that it gives them the opportunity to practice the breathe in – move arms up as you exhale – breathe in, breathe out, breathe in, exhale and bring your body back to earth with your hands by your side.

As we have previously explained the breathing and the movements are exceptionally important and the harmony that is linked between your breathing and the movements means that you are letting the flow go through your energy points and that's what yoga aims to do. A variation on this pose is that you place your foot against your thigh and balance on one leg. Then, let that leg down to the mat and use the other. Remember, breathe in move the leg, breathe out, leave it there, breathe in, breathe out and let the leg down to the floor.

The triangle pose is a good pose for beginners as well. This pose is started in a standing position with your feet reasonably far apart (about three feet). Take your arms out to the sides of you so that they are straight. Turn your left foot to about 90 degrees and then bend so that your straight arm feels its way down your leg to your ankle. This produces a triangular shape. Then do the same movement with the other leg.

Remember, all the time that your arm is reaching down toward your ankle, the other arm is reached straight out at the same angle but in an upward direction. When you reach the point that your arm is in the air and the other is on your ankle, breathe in and out and count to five overall before moving back to the central position.

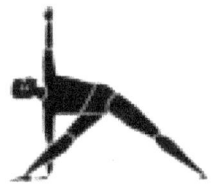

You can see by this small cartoon that you can indeed practice this even more and become more advanced at it by reaching down to the carpet behind your stretched out leg but don't try this until you are comfortable with it. This all strengthens the core of the body and helps mobility but you don't need to do the exercise to the extent that it hurts you or causes problems with your mobility. Take it slowly and be happy with the progress you are permitted to make if you have mobility problems and following the breathing exercises will help you to obtain even more movement and to get a little further with the movement next time.

The Cobra Pose is a great one for newbies as well because it doesn't require you to try anything that it too painful for your body. Lie on your mat face downward this time with your feet stretched out behind you. Place your thumbs by the side of your hips and use your hands to pull up the front of your body. Pull in the pelvic area of your body and straighten the upper part of your back at the same time. Make sure that your head is straight and that your shoulders are used to push down away from your head toward the mat. Raise your chest and feel the burn. This exercise is great for the core and for the pelvic area but it's one that will help you with your posture as well.

Chapter 20: Includes An In-Depth Self-Treatment Meditation.

To Begin Self-Treatment

Giving a self-treatment will take anywhere from a few minutes to an hour or more. You will be guided in how much time you need. Go through all the hand positions for a full-body treatment. Find a relaxing, quiet place where you can be comfortable and uninterrupted, preferably lying down or sitting in a comfortable position. However, if you cannot find that quiet, comfortable place, it is better to do Reiki wherever and whenever you can, than not at all – at the movies, on the bus, in a waiting room, etc. The benefit of Reiki is that it is available wherever you are! Do not let location stop you. However, if possible, give yourself the gift of a calming, relaxing place to practice self-treatment and self-care. You may feel

Reiki more freely when you are in a calm, meditative state, however it is not necessary, as Reiki will flow through you merely from intent.

Note: If during the self-treatment you do not feel Reiki flowing freely, begin abdominal breathing for a few moments to help the flow of energy.

The hand positions are for general guidance. You may add or remove hand positions as you gain experience, or as your intuition guides you. Dr. Usui initially taught in this way – using intuition to place hands where you were guided to. Later, Reiki evolved to include specific hand positions. Many practitioners find that by treating all the positions, i.e. "the whole body" you will be able to treat the disease and not just the symptoms. Therefore, you may be guided to treat all the positions, and then treat specific locations. As you grow in your practice you will find a method that works, indeed, the method may change with each treatment. However, as a beginner it is recommended to include all the positions in your treatments.

Your Hands

Wash your hands.

Remove any jewelry.

During Reiki treatments it is important to keep your fingers together (with no space between them) to allow the Reiki energy to flow freely from your hands.

Meditate

Begin the Reiki session by holding your palms together in the prayer position directly in front of your chest. Center your thoughts on Reiki healing energy and give yourself the intent to heal and to be healed.

Conclusion

The Sanskrit word Chakra is truly deciphered as "wheel" or "turning" and even though it began in Hindu writings, is found in the Tibetan, Chinese, and Tamil dialects also. The Chakras are vortices, which exist in our bodies and are in charge of various parts of our lives, and even though different frameworks and numbers exist, the most notable of them perceive seven noteworthy such vitality focuses.

In the Hindi writings, known as Tantras, the Chakras are portrayed as Padaka-Pancake and Sat-Cakra-Nirupama and are portions of a perplexing framework, which incorporates the Kundalini also. A considerable lot of these old writings have various varieties, posting somewhere in the range of five to twelve fundamental Padaka-Pancakes, yet every one of these frameworks has a similar objective - the enlivening of the Kundalini through the ascent of the Chakras. As the Kundalini stirs and ascends through our bodies, it continues puncturing the distinctive vortices, and the individual accomplishes another degree of Siddhi or flawlessness. A definitive objective of mindfulness is performed when the Kundalini achieves the head, and the individual is joined with the Divine.

Aside from the seven major Chakras, littler ones, which are called medians, exist also: when any of Chakras are not adjusted, at that point the individual could experience the ill effects of physical or dysfunctional behavior or irregularity. The arrangement and the enlivening of these vortices could be accomplished by the feeling of touch, which is the thing that makes the Tantric back rubs so advantageous. When you wind up in the hands of a Tantric Goddess, you won't just shape a new bond and get a very sexy back rub, yet additionally, acquire the full recuperating advantages too. Since the Universal vitality, love, and learning course through our bodies, enabling them to pass uninhibitedly and easily is significant for each part of our lives.

Thoroughly understanding this mind-boggling theory or being a dedicated adherent could bring numerous incredible advantages. However, you could utilize the Tantric back rubs, procedures, or techniques to accomplish agreement and inward harmony regardless of whether you are not by any means acquainted with the otherworldly side of this awesome educating and life reasoning.

www.ingramcontent.com/pod-product-compliance
Lightning Source LLC
Chambersburg PA
CBHW072008070526
44583CB00015B/1393